Overcoming Common Problems Series

Coping with Snoring and Sleep Apnoea
Jill Eckersley

Coping with Stomach Ulcers
Dr Tom Smith

Coping with Strokes
Dr Tom Smith

Coping with Suicide
Maggie Helen

Coping with Teenagers
Sarah Lawson

Coping with Thrush
Caroline Clayton

Coping with Thyroid Problems
Dr Joan Gomez

Curing Arthritis – The Drug-Free Way
Margaret Hills

Curing Arthritis – More Ways to a Drug-Free Life
Margaret Hills

Curing Arthritis Diet Book
Margaret Hills

Curing Arthritis Exercise Book
Margaret Hills and Janet Horwood

Cystic Fibrosis – A Family Affair
Jane Chumbley

Depression at Work
Vicky Maud

Depressive Illness
Dr Tim Cantopher

Effortless Exercise
Dr Caroline Shreeve

Fertility
Julie Reid

The Fibromyalgia Healing Diet
Christine Craggs-Hinton

Garlic
Karen Evennett

Getting a Good Night's Sleep
Fiona Johnston

The Good Stress Guide
Mary Hartley

Heal the Hurt: How to Forgive and Move On
Dr Ann Macaskill

Heart Attacks – Prevent and Survive
Dr Tom Smith

Helping Children Cope with Attention Deficit Disorder
Dr Patricia Gilbert

Helping Children Cope with Bullying
Sarah Lawson

Helping Children Cope with Change and Loss
Rosemary Wells

Helping Children Cope with Divorce
Rosemary Wells

Helping Children Cope with Grief
Rosemary Wells

Helping Children Cope with Stammering
Jackie Turnbull and Trudy Stewart

Helping Children Get the Most from School
Sarah Lawson

How to Accept Yourself
Dr Windy Dryden

How to Be Your Own Best Friend
Dr Paul Hauck

How to Cope with Anaemia
Dr Joan Gomez

How to Cope with Bulimia
Dr Joan Gomez

How to Cope with Stress
Dr Peter Tyrer

How to Enjoy Your Retirement
Vicky Maud

How to Improve Your Confidence
Dr Kenneth Hambly

How to Keep Your Cholesterol in Check
Dr Robert Povey

How to Lose Weight Without Dieting
Mark Barker

How to Make Yourself Miserable
Dr Windy Dryden

How to Pass Your Driving Test
Donald Ridland

How to Stand up for Yourself
Dr Paul Hauck

How to Stick to a Diet
Deborah Steinberg and Dr Windy Dryden

How to Stop Worrying
Dr Frank Tallis

The How to Study Book
Alan Brown

How to Succeed as a Single Parent
Carole Baldock

How to Untangle Your Emotional Knots
Dr Windy Dryden and Jack Gordon

Hysterectomy
Suzie Hayman

Is HRT Right for You?
Dr Anne MacGregor

Overcoming Common Problems Series

COPING WITH DYSPRAXIA

JILL ECKERSLEY is a freelance writer with many years' experience of writing on health topics. She is a regular contributor to women's and general-interest magazines, including *Good Health*, *Bella*, *Ms London*, *Goodtimes*, *Slimming World* and other titles. *Coping with Snoring and Sleep Apnoea* and *Coping with Childhood Asthma*, two books written by Jill for Sheldon Press, were both published in 2003. She lives beside the Regent's Canal in north

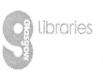
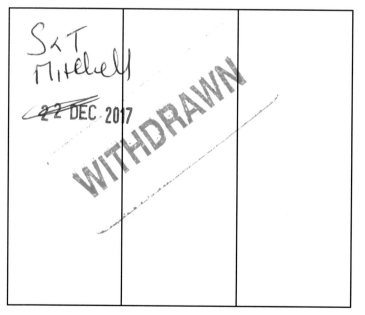

Overcoming Common Problems Series

Selected titles

A full list of titles is available from Sheldon Press,
1 Marylebone Road, London NW1 4DU, and on our website at
www.sheldonpress.co.uk

Assertiveness: Step by Step
Dr Windy Dryden and Daniel Constantinou

Body Language at Work
Mary Hartley

Cancer – A Family Affair
Neville Shone

The Cancer Guide for Men
Helen Beare and Neil Priddy

The Candida Diet Book
Karen Brody

The Chronic Fatigue Healing Diet
Christine Craggs-Hinton

Cider Vinegar
Margaret Hills

Comfort for Depression
Janet Horwood

Confidence Works
Gladeana McMahon

Considering Adoption?
Sarah Biggs

Coping Successfully with Hay Fever
Dr Robert Youngson

Coping Successfully with Pain
Neville Shone

Coping Successfully with Panic Attacks
Shirley Trickett

Coping Successfully with Prostate Cancer
Dr Tom Smith

Coping Successfully with Prostate Problems
Rosy Reynolds

Coping Successfully with RSI
Maggie Black and Penny Gray

Coping Successfully with Your Hiatus Hernia
Dr Tom Smith

Coping When Your Child Has Special Needs
Suzanne Askham

Coping with Alopecia
Dr Nigel Hunt and Dr Sue McHale

Coping with Anxiety and Depression
Shirley Trickett

Coping with Blushing
Dr Robert Edelmann

Coping with Bronchitis and Emphysema
Dr Tom Smith

Coping with Candida
Shirley Trickett

Coping with Childhood Asthma
Jill Eckersley

Coping with Chronic Fatigue
Trudie Chalder

Coping with Coeliac Disease
Karen Brody

Coping with Cystitis
Caroline Clayton

Coping with Depression and Elation
Dr Patrick McKeon

Coping with Eczema
Dr Robert Youngson

Coping with Endometriosis
Jo Mears

Coping with Epilepsy
Fiona Marshall and
Dr Pamela Crawford

Coping with Fibroids
Mary-Claire Mason

Coping with Gallstones
Dr Joan Gomez

Coping with a Hernia
Dr David Delvin

Coping with Incontinence
Dr Joan Gomez

Coping with Long-Term Illness
Barbara Baker

Coping with the Menopause
Janet Horwood

Coping with Polycystic Ovary Syndrome
Christine Craggs-Hinton

Coping with Psoriasis
Professor Ronald Marks

Coping with Rheumatism and Arthritis
Dr Robert Youngson

Coping with SAD
Fiona Marshall and Peter Cheevers

Overcoming Common Problems

Coping with Dyspraxia

Jill Eckersley

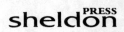
sheldon **PRESS**

First published in Great Britain in 2004 by
Sheldon Press
1 Marylebone Road
London NW1 4DU

British Library Cataloguing-in-Publication Data

A catalogue record for this book is available from the British Library

ISBN 0–85969–920–X

1 3 5 7 9 10 8 6 4 2

Typeset by Deltatype Limited, Birkenhead, Wirral
Printed in Great Britain by Biddles Ltd
www.biddles.co.uk

Contents

Acknowledgements

I would not have been able to write this book without the expertise of the Dyspraxia Foundation, whose small staff were unfailingly helpful and more than generous with their time. Thanks are also due to the many experts I spoke to, notably educational psychologist Madeleine Portwood, Dr Amanda Kirby of the Dyscovery Centre in Cardiff, physiotherapist Michele Lee, occupational therapist Therese Jackson, speech therapist Pam Williams, research psychologist Margaret Cousins and Professor Neil Marlow of Queen's Medical Centre in Nottingham.

My most grateful thanks, however, go to the many people living with dyspraxia every day who were willing to talk to me about their own experiences of growing up with what was, until very recently, a little-understood difficulty – and, of course, the parents who are now fighting for proper treatment and facilities for youngsters coping with dyspraxia today. Special thanks are also due to Mary Colley of the Adult Dyspraxia Support Group.

1
What is Dyspraxia?

Dyspraxia is not the easiest of conditions to define. The Dyspraxia Foundation, which is campaigning for more research, better treatment and more understanding of the problems it causes, calls it 'an impairment, or immaturity, of the organization of movement'. It is thought that as many as one in ten people may suffer from it to some degree, and about 2 per cent of the population is seriously affected, yet most people have never heard of it.

The fact that it is a hidden handicap – you can't immediately see that someone has dyspraxia the way you can see that someone has Down's Syndrome or is a wheelchair user – is part of the problem. Until recently, many cases were misdiagnosed or not diagnosed at all. Children with dyspraxia were dismissed as naughty or clumsy. Indeed. 'Clumsy Child Syndrome' was one of the earlier names for the condition, which has been known and recognized, though not always effectively managed, through most of the twentieth century.

Other names you might come across for dyspraxia are Developmental Co-ordination Disorder, Minimal Brain Dysfunction, Motor Learning Difficulty or Perpetuo-Motor Dysfunction – none of which exactly trip off the tongue! Some experts and parents are not happy with the 'dyspraxic' label either, as it doesn't really express the range of problems suffered by people with the condition. They feel that it is more important to find appropriate therapy for the practical difficulties faced by each individual – playing sport, organizing their life, remembering instructions or speaking clearly – than it is to find the right 'label' for them.

Dyspraxia is associated with 'movement difficulty' and clumsiness, though this is only part of the story. Children with dyspraxia are, typically, those who are never picked for team games because they have difficulty throwing and catching a ball. Their movements are often awkward and uncoordinated, and their 'spatial awareness' is poor. They may blunder around barging into people, or stand much too close to others when they want to attract their attention or talk to them.

'If there's one small brick in a large playground, he will fall over it,' is how one parent expressed it.

Babies affected by the condition may initially just be thought to be slightly late developers. They are often late reaching their milestones, like crawling, walking or feeding themselves. Toddlers find it hard to master skills like dressing themselves, eating with a knife and fork, or walking up and down stairs. School-age children may have trouble with handwriting, copying from the blackboard, following complex instructions, and generally getting themselves organized. Because dyspraxia is about the *organization* of movement, and not just movement itself, there are often associated problems with perception, thought, speech and language. People with dyspraxia don't always understand the messages conveyed by their senses, or how to translate those messages into action. As an example, they may misread the sort of visual or auditory cues the rest of us take for granted. Children in a busy classroom or adults in an open-plan office might find it hard to pick out the 'important' sounds from the general background buzz – so they may be accused of not listening, or not concentrating. Judging time, space and distance is hard for them, which is why many adult dyspraxics have problems learning to drive and some never master it. Even simple household tasks like pouring water from kettle to teapot or opening a can may be difficult for them. Telling left from right and front from back is another problem, as is negotiating spaces and walking up and down stairs or stepping off kerbs.

Social skills

Social skills can be a problem too. Children with dyspraxia may seem young for their years or, alternatively, be happier in the company of adults. They may be unable to work out from someone's facial expression whether she is angry, sad or frustrated. They then react in an inappropriate way, which can lead to misunderstandings. Planning and organizing thought may also be hard for them. For instance, many people with dyspraxia find it very difficult to follow a series of instructions, preferring to do one thing at a time. This means that something which sounds quite simple, like going to the Post Office, weighing a parcel, buying the right stamps and posting the parcel, is hard for them. Typically they might follow the first instruction and the last, omitting the steps in between.

Speech

Some children with dyspraxia may be late talkers, or their early speech may be very hard to understand because they can't make the precise movements of mouth, throat and tongue necessary to produce intelligible speech. This condition is called developmental verbal dyspraxia, and is normally treated by speech and language therapists.

'Developmental verbal dyspraxia is a type of speech disorder,' says Pam Williams, Principal Speech and Language Therapist at the Nuffield Hearing and Speech Centre in London.

> The core problem these children have is their inability to co-ordinate movement. This may affect their hands, legs, body – or the apparatus which produces speech. Between 5 and 8 per cent of the school population has speech and language difficulties, and a percentage of those will have developmental verbal dyspraxia. About half of the children we treat have other dyspraxias as well – in other words, they have additional co-ordination difficulties – and a half don't.

Treating children with developmental verbal dyspraxia is a specialized job, and speech therapists refer children to the Nuffield Centre for a second opinion.

'What everyone can recognize is that these children's speech is unintelligible, and outside the range we expect for their age,' Pam says.

> Many can only make a small range of sounds, have trouble with both consonants and vowels, can't combine consonants and vowels together, and have even more problems with long words – for instance they can say 'cat' but not 'caterpillar'. The most important thing is to make sure they get some therapy. Developmental verbal dyspraxia is treated slightly differently from other speech problems, with more emphasis on the actual *production* of

sounds, but any speech therapy is better than none! It can take time, but generally the prognosis is good.

Parents of the children I see say that their children have always been difficult to understand. It's acceptable for a 2-year-old to say 'tat' instead of 'cat' but more worrying in a 5-year-old. We do treat children as young as 3, right up to the teens.

Children with dyspraxia face two sets of problems. The first includes the practical difficulties of not being able to do all the things their peers can do – from buttoning their coats to playing football. The other problems are the psychological ones, being labelled 'difficult' or 'stupid' or 'slow' when they may, of course, be none of those things. Many children with dyspraxia grow up with low self-esteem because they are left out of their peers' activities and never seem to be good at anything that matters. They are sometimes bullied because they are seen to be different.

Awareness

Lack of awareness of the condition among the general public, and even among professionals in health and education, causes problems for families with a dyspraxic child. A survey of parents by the Dyspraxia Foundation in the mid-1990s revealed what they describe as 'a worrying tendency by men, particularly those in positions of authority, either to lay the blame on the mother for the child's difficulties, or to discount her concerns'. Several parents we interviewed for this book ruefully described being stigmatized as a 'neurotic mum' when they expressed concern that their child did not seem to be able to keep up with his or her peer group.

One of the aims of the Dyspraxia Foundation, the charity set up in 1987 as the Dyspraxia Trust by two mothers who had met at Great Ormond Street Hospital, is to promote awareness and understanding of the condition, so that old-fashioned attitudes like those described above don't add to the difficulties faced by those affected by the condition.

Dyspraxia is not a condition that you necessarily grow out of. Some people do find that their co-ordination improves as they get older; others don't. Some dyspraxic children become dyspraxic adults, who then have difficulties of their own. Driving a car, distinguishing left from right, even using simple gadgets like a corkscrew or tin-opener, can all pose problems for them.

'I didn't find out that I had dyspraxia until I was in my late thirties,' Elizabeth says.

> At school I was very isolated and often bullied. I was hopeless at sport and always the last to be picked for the team. I didn't learn to read until I was ten and couldn't do maths either. I was just regarded as lazy or stupid or careless most of the time.
>
> I did manage to pass my exams and go on to study history at university but had trouble in the world of work. I became a librarian, but my short-term memory problems meant that I made mistakes in filing and eventually was asked to leave my job.
>
> Relationships have never been easy for me either. I have always been very straightforward and bad at interpreting the unwritten rules – I couldn't cope with office politics, for instance. And I have never been able to learn to drive, which is probably just as well as I'm sure I would be a danger on the road.
>
> I did marry and have a family but found having and bringing up my children very stressful. In labour I found it hard to 'push' properly, or cope with gas-and-air. I was no good at domestic things like cooking or even childcare.
>
> It wasn't until I met a friend who was a physiotherapist and she told me I sounded as if I had dyspraxia that it all started to make sense. Eventually I was properly assessed by a psychologist and a physiotherapist, and had help with everyday tasks from two very good occupational therapists.
>
> Even the simplest tasks don't come naturally to me, but I now find that if I write down what I have to do, breaking it down into small steps, I can manage much better. I'm 43 now and welcome the increased awareness of dyspraxia, especially in schools and colleges. But we still have a long way to go before everyone knows what dyspraxia is and that it isn't something you grow out of.'

There is no cure for dyspraxia at present, although some children find that they are better able to cope as they get older. However, the condition can be managed, with appropriate treatment from a 'team' of therapists. People with dyspraxia can learn better physical co-ordination if they practise special exercises, having been taught by a physiotherapist. They can learn to organize their lives better with practical help from an occupational therapist. Those who have problems with speech and language can be referred for help to a speech and language therapist. Parents, carers, schools and colleges can all play a part in helping people with dyspraxia to feel included. Counselling or psychotherapy may be offered if appropriate.

Early diagnosis

It is generally thought to be important that dyspraxia is diagnosed as early as possible so that a child's specialist educational and social needs can be identified and treated. Paediatric physiotherapist Michele Lee, who specializes in the treatment of dyspraxia, says that the condition, if undiagnosed, will affect a child's intellectual, social and emotional development.

'Children who move confidently develop a good self-image and feel able to attempt new tasks and explore new areas without feeling threatened by failure,' she says. 'Children who don't have this often simply stop trying, and this can later lead to truancy and delinquency.'

Educational psychologist Madeleine Portwood first became interested in the subject of dyspraxia in the 1980s.

At the time, I was working with a group of children with emotional and behavioural difficulties, many of whom had been excluded from mainstream school. They were aged between 4 and 19 and we discovered that 77 per cent of them had unidentified neurological developmental disorders, including dyspraxia.

We must identify these children early because the condition has an impact, not only on their future learning, but on their whole lives. In 1996 I took part in a BBC documentary about young offenders where about 50 per cent of them had dyspraxia. I wanted to open up the whole subject to parents, teachers and the wider community and show that low-level intervention for 4- to 6-year-olds could prevent so many serious problems in later life. Therapy sessions can help, but the focus must be on normalization so that these children are better understood. Their needs must be catered for, so that they can be accommodated in mainstream schools.

In a study in 1997, the Dyspraxia Foundation found that many parents were aware that their child had a problem by the age of about 3, but that dyspraxia was often not diagnosed until the child was between 6 and 7 or even older.

It is sometimes not until a child goes to school that it's possible to see the difference between what he can achieve and what other children his age are doing, so that difficulties become much more obvious. Babies don't all develop at the same rate. First-time parents, especially, may have no standard of comparison and may sometimes be dismissed as over-anxious by health professionals.

Part of the problem may be that the symptoms of dyspraxia are easily confused with other developmental or behavioural disorders like dyslexia, attention deficit hyperactivity disorder (ADHD) or even Asperger's Syndrome or autism. The British Dyslexia Association's checklist includes characteristics which are also associated with dyspraxia – for instance, difficulties with orientation and direction, confusion between left and right, east and west, erratic handwriting, trouble copying down from the blackboard, clumsiness and a lack of physical co-ordination.

Some ADHD children also have dyspraxia, so getting a definite diagnosis is not always easy. Most ADHD children have problems with 'fine motor skills' like handwriting, colouring-in, and tying shoelaces. Some also lack 'gross motor skills' like running, catching a ball and riding a bicycle. Like children with dyspraxia they tend to barge around bumping into things and falling over, so it isn't always easy for even experts to tell the difference. However, not all children with dyspraxia are hyperactive.

Meg's daughter Chloe, now 13, has always been a quiet, 'manageable' child, though Meg began to suspect there was something wrong when she was a baby.

'She was very difficult to feed and breast-feeding was really traumatic,' she says.

Then she always had problems picking up toys, and although she did eventually crawl, it was rather late, and she was almost 2 before she walked.

One Health Visitor told me she thought Chloe might be deaf because she seemed so unresponsive, but she always got upset when an aeroplane flew over or a balloon burst at children's parties, so we knew it couldn't be that. She had three grommet operations for suspected 'glue ear' but she still didn't talk. When she was 2 and a half a speech therapist mentioned dyspraxia to me. I had never heard of it.

When Chloe first went to school she still had communication problems and poor social skills. Other children complained that she was rough and would bump into them, or 'push in' when they were playing. We did see a paediatrician who gave me useful tips like telling me to give Chloe one instruction at a time, instead of confusing her by telling her to fetch her shoes and her coat and remember to brush her teeth. Her brain just doesn't process information the way other people's brains do.

Meg has since been told that Chloe has learning difficulties as well as dyspraxia, and she has recently transferred from a mainstream school to one for children with moderate learning difficulties.

'There is no real "checklist" you can give to parents which will show that their child has dyspraxia,' comments Madeleine Portwood.

I would say that the majority – around 60 per cent – of children with dyspraxia have *some* other developmental disorders too, like ADHD, autism or dyslexia. Some children seem clumsy because they are very impulsive. A specific assessment by a specialist can identify the particular hand movements which are characteristic of dyspraxia. Individual children may have other problems too. We once researched 800 people with dyspraxia and found that 82 per cent had not gone through the crawling stage as babies. In order to crawl, a baby needs to move her right arm and her left leg and these children can't co-ordinate those movements. Young children may also have delayed speech, not because of what they're trying to say but because they can't co-ordinate the right movements of lips, tongue and soft palate.

'It hurts when your child is "different",' says Pam, whose 10-year-old son Jon has now been diagnosed with dyspraxia, ADHD and slight Asperger's Syndrome. Pam has known since Jon went to playgroup that there was something wrong, but initially she had no idea what to do or where to seek help. She admits that it has been a strain.

At one point, I had a nervous breakdown and became so frustrated that I actually hit Jon. I felt absolutely terrible about it, but luckily, I was able to ask for help from the Social Services before things got any worse. They offered me a carer for a couple of hours a week so that I could have a break, and that did help. If you have a child who is seen as difficult, other parents and children often don't want to know.

The only advice I had when he was small came from my Health Visitor, who told me I shouldn't give him a dummy!

Things started to go wrong when he went to playgroup and they couldn't control him. He is quite badly affected and lacks both gross and fine motor skills. He is also hyperactive and has speech problems. Because he couldn't do what the other children did he became very frustrated, had tantrums and hurt himself. He was still doing that when he went to primary school.

Pam and Jon had mixed experiences with both educational and health professionals.

I went to meet him from school one day. The Deputy Head brought him out and said, in front of all the other parents and children, 'We've had a terrible day with your son!' Jon was crying and I felt so humiliated. We went home and he told me he wanted to die. You can imagine how that made me feel.

Eventually we saw an educational psychologist and an occupational therapist. They were both very helpful, although there was a long waiting list for treatment. Sessions with the OT improved his throwing and catching skills, balancing and handwriting, but there's still a lot he can't do. He finds walking upstairs very difficult because there seems to be a slow link between his brain, his eyes and his legs. Once he lifts a foot he loses his balance and finds it hard to stay in control. He feels a failure because he can't ride a bike like the other kids. He's very emotional and gets upset if things aren't in their proper places, and is worried by loud

9

noises. He can't yet use a knife and fork and I still have to wipe his bottom for him.

His speech is still a problem and he can't always express what he is trying to say. He is learning to cope with money, but he still has no sense of danger and would trust anyone, which is worrying, of course.

Set against that, there are things he is good at, like history, geography and art. He loves his Play Station and knows all about cars. He says he wants to be a car designer when he grows up.

Bringing Jon up hasn't been easy for any of us. His father had dyslexia so is very understanding, but it has put a strain on our marriage. My parents still can't accept there's anything wrong with their grandson and keep telling me he will grow out of his problems.

Now that we know what's wrong with Jon we will do whatever it takes to help him lead a normal life. We are in touch with the Dyspraxia Foundation so we have met other parents and children and share coping strategies.

2

What Causes Dyspraxia?

Parents who are told their child has dyspraxia often ask about the causes. The answers doctors are able to give are often not terribly satisfactory. In spite of many years of research, not much is definitely known.

The simplest way to express what has gone wrong is that the brains of people with dyspraxia are 'wired up' slightly differently from those of the rest of us. When you think what a massively complicated structure the brain is – best seen, perhaps, as a sort of switchboard for the human communications system, and containing over 100 billion nerve cells, or 'neurons' – it's easy to see how dysfunction can happen.

Interestingly, many people with dyspraxia, particularly adults, prefer to think of the condition as simply 'different' rather than 'wrong'. They point out that they have many skills and talents and that the fact that their intelligence seems to work in a slightly different way from the majority of us can actually be an advantage, rather than a problem.

How the brain works

The **central nervous system** consists of the brain and spinal cord.

The **peripheral nervous system** has three parts. One extends throughout the body to the skin and muscles. Another links the brain to the senses – eyes, ears, nose and taste buds. The third, known as the **autonomic nervous system**, controls our involuntary body functions like breathing and digestion. Different parts of the brain itself control different functions in the body – for instance vision, heart rate, emotions or balance.

Information is carried throughout the nervous system by electrical impulses and chemical messengers called neurotransmitters. Electrical impulses carry signals along the neurons themselves. Chemical neurotransmitters carry signals across the gaps between neurons. They are released from one neuron to bind with the receptor sites of the next. When nerve cells are immature, under-active, over-active or poorly co-ordinated, brain disorders occur. For example, epilepsy is caused by electrical disturbances of certain nerve cells. Parkinson's disease is caused by lack of a neurotransmitter called dopamine. Children with ADHD have been found to have lower levels of both dopamine and another neurotransmitter, noradrenaline.

It is not yet known whether dyspraxia is caused by faults in the cells themselves or in the gaps between them, known as synapses, or possibly even by lack of certain neurotransmitters, the brain's chemical messengers. Because children with dyspraxia present with a variety of different symptoms, and because the condition so often overlaps with other developmental disorders like ADHD, dyslexia and Asperger's Syndrome, it is difficult to say with certainty exactly which part of the brain is involved in a particular individual. Some experts say the problem is in the cerebellum – an area which affects balance and involuntary movement. This is called the 'cerebellar deficit hypothesis'. However, other experts feel that as not all those with dyspraxia have balance problems, other areas of the brain may also be involved.

'It's a very complex picture and no one explanation seems to fit in every case,' explains research psychologist Margaret Cousins. 'When someone has a stroke, you can often see which area of the brain is involved, but this just isn't possible with dyspraxia.'

According to the Dyspraxia Foundation, dyspraxia is said to be the result of an immaturity in the development of the neurons or nerve cells in the brain, rather than brain damage. For most people with the condition, there is no obvious cause. There are many suggestions as to why this might have occurred – perhaps lack of oxygen at a crucial period in pregnancy, or even a viral infection at the time, around the fifth week, when the baby's nervous system is beginning to form. A genetic element may be involved. There could be an inherited tendency in the family towards similar neurological disorders.

Premature babies

Researchers have looked at the factors in pregnancy which seem to be implicated in developmental disorders. There does seem to be a link with babies born prematurely, or 'small for dates', which, in their turn, are influenced by factors like smoking and poor diet in mothers-to-be.

Professor Neil Marlow of Queen's Medical Centre in Nottingham is a neonatologist with a special interest in the progress of premature babies as they grow up, especially in their motor problems, which can be significant. He says that, so far, the 'cause' of dyspraxia remains unclear. For example, although many premature babies seem to develop motor problems as well as conditions like ADHD, by no means all children with dyspraxia were premature babies.

'We have studied the reasons why motor problems might develop in these children, and looked at a possible association with brain injury,' he says.

> Premature babies are at risk of bleeding injury or oxygen starvation at birth and we can pick this up with ultrasound. We thought this might lead to later dyspraxia, but it doesn't seem to do so. The brain seems to be able to compensate during a period of very fast growth, such as occurs around the time of birth.
>
> Magnetic resonance imaging and associated technologies show us that pre-term babies do have slightly different brains. They are less folded and have less supporting tissue. It is possible that early birth disturbs the trajectory of brain growth. In the early years, we make millions of connections between the neurons in our brains, and then we lose a lot of them, only keeping those which have proved useful. It's possible that babies born prematurely may have fewer brain connections to choose from, so they don't necessarily choose the best ones.
>
> Basically, though, we don't yet know exactly what happens in the brains of people with dyspraxia. In a very small number of cases we can say why the condition developed but in most cases we can't give a reason. It is likely to be a complex problem and we don't yet know which area, or areas, of the brain are affected or what part genetics plays.

It seems to be fairly well established that premature babies are more at risk of developing dyspraxia, but as yet all the causes of prematurity are not known either.

Metabolism

Researchers are also looking at the part metabolism plays in dyspraxia, since many children with the condition (about one-third according to a recent University of Oxford/Durham LEA study) seem to have a problem breaking down essential fatty acids. There is some evidence that essential fatty acid supplements can play a part in the successful management of dyspraxia in some people, though this doesn't appear to work for everyone. (See Chapter 8 for details.) Babies who are breast-fed for longer get more essential fatty acids from mother's milk and are less likely to suffer from developmental disorders.

Babies are born with a limited, but fairly sophisticated, range of movements. Even newborns will grasp a finger and hold on tight! Dyspraxia expert and educational psychologist Madeleine Portwood explains that a baby's brain adapts to its environment through a process of natural selection. When the messages transmitted between nerve cells produce a successful outcome, like grasping a finger or a toy, the connections used to achieve that outcome will be reinforced while others, which have not been used, may disappear.

'In the case of the dyspraxic child, the reinforced interconnections between nerve cells in the brain are reduced in number,' she says. In other words, some of the brain cells remain immature.

Research into the mechanisms – either neurological or metabolic – which cause dyspraxia is still going on. Meanwhile, it seems more important for those affected that the problem is identified as early as possible and that they are given appropriate treatment in order to help them cope with everyday life.

3

Dyspraxia and the Pre-School Child

All babies and children develop at different rates, and health professionals usually advise parents, 'not to worry, he'll catch up' if their child seems to be a late developer. Dyspraxia is a condition that isn't always obvious in babyhood, especially if the child is only mildly affected. However, looking back, parents of dyspraxic children often say that deep down, they had the feeling that things were not as they should be. First-time parents, though, often have no standards of comparison, and are not sure what their baby *should* be able to do at a particular age. Even experienced parents like Janey, whose youngest daughter Louise was diagnosed with dyspraxia at 6, found it hard at first to pinpoint what was wrong.

'I have two older children but even so I found that I had forgotten exactly what they were like at Louise's age,' she says.

I think the first thing I noticed was that Lou was a very jumpy and nervous baby. She didn't just start at loud noises, but even when she saw I was looking at her. She didn't like bright lights, and was a poor sleeper who had to be swathed in blankets before she would go to sleep at all.

When she started to walk I could see there was something not quite right. She would walk on tiptoe, which meant that she fell forward a lot. Her gait was awkward, with her legs wide apart as if she was steadying herself all the time.

Like many parents, Janey found that Louise's difficulties became much more obvious when she went to nursery school.

Even though I used to be a nurse, I had never heard of dyspraxia. I couldn't work out what was wrong with my daughter. She seemed to be of normal intelligence and had an excellent vocabulary. On the other hand, it took her ages even to attempt to dress herself and she couldn't tie her shoelaces. When the other children at nursery picked up pencils or crayons and drew figures and houses, Lou just couldn't do anything like that. Her walking was very odd, as I said, and I noticed that as she walked, her arms seemed to mirror what her legs were doing. She had a few speech problems, too, but when we were referred for speech therapy, the therapist told us that her problems were so mild that she would probably grow out of them.

Pre-school children with dyspraxia show a whole range of developmental problems which often makes it difficult to arrive at a definite diagnosis. Some babies, for instance, are a problem to feed. Meg, for example, remembers trying to breast-feed her daughter Chloe as

a complete nightmare. I had to have a lot of help from my Health Visitor. As Chloe grew, her other problems became obvious too. She couldn't pick her toys up and was very late in both crawling and walking. She was almost 2 before she walked. She wasn't a very responsive baby and when she didn't babble as most babies do, I was told that she might be deaf. I didn't think that this could be the case as she did respond to some sounds and could always make me understand what she wanted by pointing!

Pam's son Jon, who has subsequently been diagnosed with dyspraxia, ADHD and slight Asperger's, was also, as Pam says, a 'difficult' baby.

He was born feet first and I had to have an emergency Caesarian. He was also born with the cord wrapped round his neck. As a small baby he didn't seem able to suck properly. First I tried breast-feeding him, and then I tried bottles with different-sized teats. Nothing helped, and he cried constantly. I walked the streets at night with him but he seemed to be soothed only by the sound of the washing-machine!

He was difficult to wean on to solid food and couldn't cope with anything chewy. I had to mash his food up for ages. I didn't worry too much when he was late reaching his milestones, but there were things I noticed, like he could never crawl but would shuffle along on his bottom, and he couldn't drive his little pedal car. When friends brought their children round Jon would play alongside them but not with them.

I thought he was just a bit slow and would catch up. When he first went to nursery, they asked me if he had hearing problems. He didn't seem to listen to what was said to him and at story-time they had to hold him down! He fell over so often he looked like a battered child.

He was given a hearing test, but it wasn't until we moved to a different area and he started primary school that we got an appointment with an educational psychologist.

The Dyspraxia Foundation has produced a checklist of symptoms which might indicate dyspraxia in a pre-school child. Such children, they say,

- reach their milestones later than other children – they are slow to roll over, sit, stand, walk and talk. Many dyspraxic children never crawl at all, though some do;
- have difficulty with physical movement, finding it hard to run, hop, skip, jump, catch or kick a ball as well as other children of their age;
- have trouble making and keeping friends and are poor at judging how to behave in the company of other people;
- don't really understand concepts like 'in', 'on', 'in front of', 'behind' and so on;
- often have difficulty walking up and down stairs;
- are poor at dressing themselves, struggling with buttons and other fastenings;
- are slow and hesitant in most of their actions;
- find it hard to learn anything instinctively, but have to be taught basic skills;
- fall over a lot;
- are not very good at holding pencils, crayons or paint brushes;
- are poor at jigsaws or shape-sorting games;
- produce only very immature artwork;
- lack concentration, and are often anxious and easily distracted.

Parents of dyspraxic children mention all kinds of other problems which seem to be characteristic of the condition, like feeding difficulties. Either the child has always been difficult to feed, or they will only accept a highly restricted diet, or they seem to tolerate certain foods very poorly – for instance, dairy products. They are also poor sleepers on the whole, and seem constantly 'on the go' even though their movements are often uncoordinated so that they find it hard to pedal a bike, for example.

'Nervous' problems, like an extreme sensitivity to loud noises or bright lights, are also often mentioned.

Sadly, dyspraxic children are sometimes made to feel left out and 'different' even at the nursery-school stage. Because their behaviour can be erratic, other children don't want to play with them, so they tend to be left on their own. Staff at nurseries and playgroups may find them 'difficult' as they tend to be excitable, hard to control, loud, easily upset, and liable to temper tantrums, often caused by pure frustration.

Helpful strategies

The fact that children can begin to have problems so early underlines what the experts say – the younger the child is when they are diagnosed, the better. All the problems faced by dyspraxic toddlers can be addressed by appropriate therapy, careful management and common-sense tips and hints from other parents. For instance, once you know your child finds it hard to follow a series of instructions like 'put the cup on the table in the kitchen' you can break the instruction down into its component parts in a way which the child can follow.

It has been suggested that a more traditional style of parenting may benefit young children with dyspraxia. For example, an old-fashioned 'baby-walker' with a bar-type handle and bricks can help them to walk properly. Rolling about on the floor, starting from a prone (on the tummy) position, can help strengthen the neck muscles and prepare for crawling. Lots of directed activity, with games and nursery-rhymes which involve actions, will improve co-ordination in a way that watching the TV or video does not. Sitting round the table for family meals teaches uncoordinated children how to use a knife and fork, which helps co-ordination as well as table manners!

Playgroups and nurseries

When children go to playgroup or nursery they may find a very 'busy' or lively atmosphere distracting or distressing. And you only have to imagine how it must feel to be the odd one out, the one who *never* wins the game, the one who is always last to complete even a simple task, to see where self-esteem problems begin. It's no wonder that children with undiagnosed dyspraxia are often seen as troublesome, uncontrollable or over-anxious.

At present, the general feeling seems to be that children with 'special needs' should be integrated into everyday life, which includes daycare and pre-school provision. Childminders, nursery schools and playgroups are all more open-minded than they once were – though you may still find that many individuals haven't heard of dyspraxia! A spokeswoman for the National Childminding Association was not familiar with the condition, but told me that in her long experience, childminders were willing to care for all kinds of children, from those who use wheelchairs to deaf children and those with cerebral palsy. Many were willing to take on extra training so that they could learn sign language, for example, or find out more about medication if they were going to care for a toddler affected by diabetes or asthma.

'I would recommend that parents be completely open and transparent with their prospective childminder,' she said.

It's all about parents and childminders working together to help and support one another in doing their best for the child. Childminders often have experience of looking after children with special needs, not only for working parents but also for the Social Services. If they haven't come across a particular condition before they will probably ask the parents to tell them all about it and explain exactly what their child needs and what his difficulties are.

Inclusion is also the policy of the Pre-School Learning Alliance (PSLA). Their Special Needs Officer, Nicky Young, who is herself the mother of a son with dyspraxia, says that they are currently re-evaluating their training courses so that playgroup leaders know about the whole range of 'special needs' and how all children can be catered for in a pre-school setting. As she points out,

Many children are not diagnosed until they are older, though. We have also found that playgroup leaders are nervous of 'getting it wrong' as there seems to be a lot to learn about the Disability

19

Discrimination Act and the Special Needs Code of Practice. However, we say that if the attitude is right and staff are willing to talk to parents and find out what the child's needs are, things tend to work out.

We have certainly moved on since my son was small and was put into 'remedial' classes because dyspraxia just wasn't recognized.

The PSLA's literature on 'Inclusion in pre-school settings' includes information on dyspraxia for playgroup leaders and keyworkers. They suggest working with parents, and with health professionals like occupational therapists (OTs) if the child has been diagnosed, and making sure that children

- experience success – perhaps by helping them to complete tasks they find difficult, which motivates them to try again next time;
- get lots of practice in activities and movements which don't come as naturally to them as they do to unaffected children, giving them extra time if necessary;
- take part in games and activities to help balance and co-ordination – threading, lacing, dressing dolls, jigsaws, screwing on and taking off lids, and games and rhymes involving 'actions'.

They also recommend detailed record-keeping so that the child's progress is carefully monitored.

Parents for Inclusion

For eighteen years, the campaigning group Parents for Inclusion has been working to integrate children with any kind of impairment into mainstream education, from the early years onward. They are also supported by adults with disabilities, many of whom were educated in the days when 'special schools' were the norm. Their lobbying has contributed to the latest Disability Discrimination Act and the most recent Education Act. They feel that early years provision has made great strides recently.

'It isn't very long since it was felt that special-needs children who were a bit slow or clumsy might be better catered for in special schools or separate classes, but that is no longer the case,' says Director Diana Simpson.

> Recent Government initiatives mean that every Local Education Authority, in partnership with Health, Social Services and the voluntary sector, has a remit to make sure that special-needs children are included in early years provision. As parents, we have found that many nursery teachers have flexible and open attitudes anyway and that nursery schools already think of themselves as providing for the whole community. The Government's 'Sure Start' project is especially aimed at helping disadvantaged children – including those with disabilities – and there is a real sense of energy in early learning. The DfES even has special funding to enable children with special needs to be included in mainstream nursery provision.

If the parents of children with developmental disorders like dyspraxia *do* have problems with their child's playgroup or nursery, Parents for Inclusion can offer them support. Their approach is a positive one. Rather than advising parents to withdraw their child from a particular group or school, they would always suggest working with the school to find ways to include the child. They point out that the ideal carer, childminder, playgroup leader or nursery nurse will focus on what the child can do and not what he can't – 'his strengths as well as his struggles' is the way they express it.

Every Local Authority should have an 'inclusion team' or an area Special Needs Co-ordinator (SENCO) whose job it is to make sure that all providers of early years education are working to include children with special needs.

'We work on the "social model of disability",' says a London SENCO. 'That means we look at the child's strengths and what they can do, as well as looking at where support is needed and how it can best be given.'

The SENCO will advise playgroups and nursery schools on how activities can be made accessible to all children and how children with developmental disorders like dyspraxia can be integrated, perhaps by using the child's interests to develop skills and enjoy activities she can share with the others. Even disruptive behaviour can be dealt with.

Some children react well to a short 'time out' to calm down, perhaps in a corner of the room. No eye-contact is made, so that the child doesn't feel he is getting attention for negative behaviour. Meanwhile, positive behaviour is reinforced by lots of praise. Task-specific praise works well too – saying 'you are sitting quietly, well done' rather than just 'good boy'. 'Proximity praising' is another useful technique for disruptive children. For example, at story-time when the others are all sitting quietly while one child is jumping about and shouting, you might praise the other children for sitting quietly with their arms folded. If you pay no attention at all to the disruptive one, quite often he will join the others. Even if another child says, 'Miss, Billy's running about,' you just need to say, quite calmly, 'We're not taking any notice of Billy, we're sitting down waiting for a story.' It's all about rewarding good behaviour instead of wasting time shouting at the disruptive child.

Parents, nursery teachers, carers and childminders can all benefit from this kind of simple technique for managing difficult behaviour, whether or not the child has officially been diagnosed. Parents should tell nursery staff and carers if there are events or situations which upset their child so that they can be avoided or carefully managed.

Dr Amanda Kirby, the Medical Director of the Dyscovery Centre in Cardiff, which assesses and treats children with dyspraxia, recommends plenty of 'big play' and activities which build up muscle control. These can take place in a playgroup or nursery setting, and are also often things which parents can do with their child at home. Setting up obstacle courses, playing on the floor, swimming, or 'painting' the garden fence or shed with a big paintbrush and a bucket of water can all help to develop a child's motor skills.

Anne is a special-needs teacher whose husband, son and grand-daughter all have dyspraxia. She says that there is a lot parents can do at home to help their children, whether or not they have been diagnosed.

One thing to remember is that young children with dyspraxia do need *teaching*. They don't pick up skills on their own as other children do. Simple games, like throwing and catching a ball, passing a bean-bag from hand to hand or trying to knock down plastic skittles, will all help.

One thing that dyspraxic children find difficult is something we call 'crossing the midline'. What that means is, they find it hard to do things with their right hand on the left side of the body, and vice versa. If you ask a dyspraxic child to touch their left ear with their right hand, they will have problems. You can practise this with them, over and over.

'Constancy of numbers' can often be a problem for them too. My son knew that three apples and two apples made five apples, but couldn't understand that three pears and two pears meant five pears. Number games are a good idea, so that children learn that three means three, whether we are talking about apples, or sheep, or teddies.

With my grand-daughter, we practised a lot of these skills with her at home, before she went to school, so that she was much more able to keep up with her peers. Unlike other children, she didn't learn from what she saw others doing, she had to be shown.

Getting help

If you suspect your child has dyspraxia your first step should be to go to your GP or Health Visitor and ask if you can be referred to a paediatrician or a Child Development Centre. Your child may be assessed by a psychologist, physiotherapist, speech and language therapist or occupational therapist. Any or all of these health professionals will be able to work out an appropriate therapy programme, depending on the nature of the child's symptoms.

Depending on where you live and exactly what facilities are available in your area, you will probably have to wait for an appointment with the specialist. While you wait, the Dyspraxia Foundation recommends that you write down everything about your child's behaviour and developmental problems that concerns you, at home and in playgroup or nursery school. When the specialist assesses your child, she will want to know as much as you can tell her so that she can work out an appropriate programme. Children being children, your little one will probably behave quite differently in an unfamiliar setting! You know your child best and it will help if you can remember things like your child's age when he reached developmental milestones, which activities he seems to have special difficulty with, and how he reacts to other children and adults.

The Dyspraxia Foundation reports patchy provision of help around the country. You can be lucky and find a supportive GP and paediatrician, or you might face a considerable wait.

'Some GPs have never heard of the condition and we do get calls from them, asking for information,' says a spokeswoman.

Families may also face a long wait to see a paediatrician, physio or occupational therapist. A wait of 12 to 18 months is not uncommon and is obviously not acceptable. In Scotland we have heard of children being asked to wait as long as three years. Paediatricians are not always very helpful either. One distressed mum rang us saying that she had been told her son has dyspraxia – but nothing else about the condition. Physiotherapy or occupational therapy may be recommended but without any indication of when this will happen or what is involved.

4

The Dyspraxic Child at School

The most important thing to remember is that dyspraxic children are entitled to fulfil their potential at school and receive an education which is suitable for their needs, just as other children are. Where once dyspraxic children would have been labelled slow or backward, the best schools now realize that they are as intelligent as other children – sometimes more intelligent – and that with a little extra help, and recognition of their skills and talents, they can fit perfectly well into mainstream education.

It wasn't always like that. Most adults with dyspraxia can remember a time when they were shunted into 'remedial' classes and accused of being stupid, or lazy, or not trying. These days, more effort is made to help children with developmental disorders, although getting an actual diagnosis and appropriate help can still take time.

The Special Educational Needs and Disability Act of 2001 removed the remaining barriers to inclusion in the British school system and made it a legal requirement for children with special needs to be treated as favourably as all other children. Some Local Authorities – Nottingham, Bristol and the London boroughs of Newham, Hackney, Lambeth and Richmond – have made considerable progress towards a totally inclusive education system. However, 80 per cent of Local Education Authorities report a shortage of health and social services provision, and it is still, sadly, true that the vast majority of children 'excluded' from mainstream schools have special educational needs that are not being met.

The Department for Education and Skills Publications Centre (contact details on p. 91) publishes a free handbook for parents called *Special Educational Needs, a Guide for Parents and Carers* which tells you all you need to know about obtaining a statement of special educational needs (SEN) for your child. The main points they make are that

- all children are entitled to have their needs met;
- most children will have their needs met in mainstream school;

- your views should be taken into account and the wishes of your child should be listened to;
- children with special needs should get a broad, well-balanced and relevant education.

Getting a statement

They emphasize that help for your child is a co-operative effort between you as parents, your child, his school and teachers, the Local Education Authority, and sometimes Health and Social Services, depending on the degree of disability. Sometimes the school can meet a child's special needs from within its normal resources. Sometimes the LEA will be asked to 'assess' your child's needs and/or prepare a 'statement'. This is a detailed document giving information about what the child's needs are, what special help he should get, the arrangements for setting both short- and long-term goals for your child, and the school he should go to, as well as information about any non-educational needs he might have. Statements should be reviewed every year to make sure the child's needs are still being met.

Getting the best out of a child's statement is all about communication – between parents, school, LEA, and anyone else involved. You can appeal if you don't feel the experts have got it right. Many areas have parent partnership services, which provide support and advice to parents of SEN children. Contact numbers for these are listed in the DfES booklet. The Dyspraxia Foundation (both Head Office and local groups) is also an excellent source of help.

Obtaining the right help and support for your child at school, and/or a statement, is not always easy. Many parents report having to put up something of a fight and having to wait too long for the bureaucratic process, intended to help both parents, school and child, to begin to work!

'Louise had problems from the start of her primary school days,' says Janey, her mother.

She could read fluently, but her writing and art work seemed to be two or three years behind her peers. By the time she went into Year 2, I was sure there was something wrong and went to see the

26

Headmistress. I had already been told by a paediatrician that she would grow out of her difficulties, so when I asked for additional help for her, or even a statement of special needs, I was told not to be ridiculous, she wasn't nearly bad enough for that!

I have to admit, I went home and cried. Over the months Lou seemed to be falling further and further behind and there was nothing I could do. Then I saw a TV programme about dyspraxia and as soon as I saw a child walking like Lou did, I knew what her problem was. The school nurse eventually approached me with information about 'statementing' from the Education Authority. After making a lot of fuss, I managed to get a statement for Lou.

Then her world opened up. She had a helper with her for 25 hours a week on a one-to-one basis and this made all the difference to her. When she showed signs of losing concentration, her helper would tell her what she had to do. It had always been hard for her to put her thoughts down on paper, but when her helper could write things down for her, it was fine.

I couldn't believe the difference it made to Lou. I had a happy child instead of one who was either aggressive or upset most of the time. Before she was statemented she failed at everything she tried and it affected her self-esteem really badly. Afterwards, she was able to use her vivid imagination to create stories and poems which her helper wrote down for her. She also showed a real interest in how things worked and when she took her SATS in primary school she was among the top dozen children in science.

I know how lucky we are that Lou is now getting the support she needs but I hear about so many parents having a tough time. If you give children with dyspraxia the right kind of support early on in their school career, they can do really well.

Pam and her son weren't so lucky. 'It is a constant battle,' says Pam, whose 10-year-old son Jon hasn't had his special-needs statement reviewed since he started primary school.

Jon is all right in his own environment but his fine and gross motor skills are poor, he dislikes loud noises and gets very emotional if things aren't where he expects them to be. I did have to take him out of school at one point and tried teaching him at home but it wasn't a great success. Unfortunately there is a two-year wait for occupational therapy in our area and the Local Education Authority won't fund a support worker for him. I have even approached my local MP for help and started a Saturday Club for special-needs children in the area. Jon needs to learn life skills like how to handle money. He finds both maths and English difficult, though he enjoys history, geography and art.

His school wasn't very sympathetic to his needs at all and I think this is part of the problem with having a 'hidden handicap'. The children were sent on cross-country runs and of course Jon always came in last. If he had been in a wheelchair, no one would have expected him to join in!

I now run a local group for dyspraxic children and their parents. Our next project is to try and raise money for a clinic which would offer all the help our children need, from physio and occupational therapy to speech therapy and even respite care for parents, so that they wouldn't need to travel miles to see different specialists. Parents do get angry and frustrated when their children aren't offered the right kind of support. A good school with good teachers who take a flexible approach to special-needs children can make all the difference.

The Dyspraxia Foundation offers help to both parents and teachers in helping children with dyspraxia adjust to the routines of school. Whether or not a child has actually been diagnosed, the Foundation points out that there are characteristics to look out for in the classroom. Children with dyspraxia

- trip and fall over more often than other children;
- often have poor concentration and are easily distracted from what they are doing;
- may seem impervious to dangers – jumping from the top of a piece of apparatus, or heading towards a busy road;
- alternatively, may seem extra-hesitant or fearful;
- may still have speech problems;
- have poor perceptual skills and find things like constructional toys difficult or impossible to assemble;
- hesitate over which hand to use – may use the right hand to complete a task on the right side of the body and the left hand to do so on the left side;

- find it hard to take part in throwing-and-catching games, or music-and-movement; anything that involves hand–eye co-ordination;
- find it hard to remember more than one instruction at a time;
- are often the last to dress or undress themselves for PE lessons;
- have problems with handwriting;
- seem to work much more slowly than other children;
- seem very emotional and excitable, often flapping their hands or clapping inappropriately, and becoming easily distressed if things go wrong;
- are messy eaters who have problems using a knife and fork;
- don't mix well with other children and often seem to be 'loners' within a group.

The Foundation also says that simple adjustments can be made in the classroom to accommodate the slightly different style of learning appropriate for dyspraxic children. Even something as simple as attaching paper to the desk so that the child doesn't have to hold the paper steady with one hand while trying to write or draw with the other can make quite a difference! Instructions can be given one at a time and repeated several times if necessary. Like all children, those with dyspraxia respond well to praise and encouragement.

Inclusive solutions

'In the scale of things, dyspraxia is not usually a severe or profound disability,' says educational psychologist Colin Newton. Colin, who is based in Nottingham, set up his company Inclusive Solutions with fellow-psychologist Derek Wilson two years ago. They advise and train schools, teachers, parents, Local Education Authorities and other interested parties on how to include children with special needs in mainstream school. They maintain that with the right mindset and goodwill on all sides, it shouldn't be too problematic to accommodate any child with dyspraxia.

'We have been influenced by the "Total Inclusion" movement in the USA and Canada. There, children with even the most profound learning and behavioural difficulties, including those with no movement or language, have been successfully integrated into ordinary schools,' says Colin Newton.

It doesn't make sense for children to be segregated in special schools. Why put children with the same problem all together? Even difficult or challenging behaviour can be managed if the teacher is given support. Another way of dealing with it is by the 'Circle of Friends' method, involving the other children.

Parents should be aware of the SEN Code of Practice [copies of which are available from the DfES Publications Department or website – see p. 91] which states that all children should have an Individual Education Plan or IEP, with relevant targets which reflect the child's needs. Parents need to be involved in the IEP because they know from experience how to get the best from their child.

Children with dyspraxia, like all children with special needs, should be included in all school activities, so the question should always be: what accommodation needs to be made so that this can happen? If children are not taken on school trips and so on, the school could fall foul of the Disability Discrimination Act.

Similarly, the question in school should be how children with dyspraxia can access PE lessons, handwriting lessons, whatever. There are solutions to most problems – tripod grips on pencils, the use of computer keyboards – if the will is there. Parents need to feel that the child's class teacher, Head and Special Needs Co-ordinator or SENCO are on their side.

The 'dyspraxia' label should really just be a signpost towards resources and support. The best teachers are able to see the child first and the label second; to locate the child's gifts and talents and build on those. Children with dyspraxia need a school which is able to *celebrate* 'difference' – one which isn't afraid to be open and up-front and talk about it, perhaps in Citizenship or PSHE lessons, and to use books and literature which explore the issues. A school where the uniqueness of people is celebrated will be one where children are not bullied and teased because they can't catch a ball, or because they look awkward and 'different'.

Special schools

In an ideal world, of course, children who are seen as 'different' in some way would not be bullied or made to feel left out. In the real world, parents sometimes have reservations about inclusion, for these and other reasons. Meg, whose daughter Chloe has until recently always been in mainstream school in spite of her dyspraxia and learning difficulties, has just transferred her to a special school.

'I can see that socially it's good for her to be with ordinary children, but although the mainstream school did the best it could, Chloe *never* felt that she could do things as well as the others,' she comments.

Fiona belongs to a local Parents' Group who have organized activity holidays for their dyspraxic children.

'Kerry, my daughter, is in mainstream school, but I feel that children do sometimes need to be with others with the same difficulties,' she says.

'On our weekend away, the children went horse-riding and rope-climbing, and for once it didn't matter if they couldn't get it right.

If children are to be included in ordinary schools, *everyone* – from the dinner-ladies to the other children in the class – needs to know about dyspraxia. I have managed to get a statement of special needs for Kerry and her school did help, but she still often came home in tears. I did some work with her class myself, in 'Circle Time' when the children and I sat round talking about how everyone has problems, things they can't do, and explaining what Kerry's problems were. She has built up a good network of supportive friends, but many other children aren't so lucky.

On the other hand, children with dyspraxia might not fit into a special school either. Kerry had some occupational therapy at a school for children with Asperger's Syndrome and it was soon obvious she would have been completely out of place there, too.

Finding the right school

Although everyone agrees that finding the right school for your child is crucial, there is no consensus on what sort of school that should be. At the end of the day, each child is an individual and what suits one may not suit another, even when both have been diagnosed with dyspraxia.

Some parents, for instance, feel that a more traditional style of teaching suits dyspraxic children better. Anne, whose husband is dyspraxic as well as her son and grand-daughter, made this point.

My husband was taught, as all children were in those days, in an old-fashioned classroom with desks in rows. He knew that the pencils were always kept in a tin in the same place, and at the end of the day he was expected to put his pencils in that tin. That sort of structured environment and unvarying routine seemed to suit him. Today's children are expected to learn by finding out and experimenting and that doesn't really work for dyspraxic children.

Sheila and her husband Niall have opted for a private school for their dyspraxic son Daniel for similar reasons. As she says,

It isn't so much that he is in a smaller class, it's that the school offers reasonably traditional teaching with a blackboard and a quiet atmosphere. Daniel knows it's always art on Fridays, so he has to take his art overall. He has an old-fashioned desk with a lid and he knows that's where all his belongings are. He sits at the front of the class between two quiet children, he can see the teacher, the atmosphere is calm and ordered, and homework is done on regular nights. We follow the same strategies at home with him. I pick him up from school and then he does his homework before we have tea, and after that he might go to his drama club or music lesson. He did try the Cubs but found there was too much going on and it made him anxious and distracted.

Sheila describes Daniel's year in his local state school as a disaster.

It was an open-plan classroom and Daniel just couldn't cope with all the distractions. Even ordinary children are distractible and dyspraxic ones are more so! His teacher didn't believe in having her own desk, so even she was always in a different part of the room, moving around. There was lots and lots of the children's artwork on the walls; it was lovely and bright and lively but just not the right environment for a child like Daniel.

Catherine Allen, who is the Head of the Home School in north London, a special school for children with dyslexia, dyspraxia and Asperger's Syndrome, says that while many children with these conditions can cope with mainstream school, not all can.

It all depends on the child. Parents usually want mainstream school to work, but sometimes it just doesn't. Children who are bullied or socially excluded by their peers come here. We are a small school with a one to four staff/child ratio so our staff know their children very well, much better than they would be able to in a larger school. Here, no child is 'different' or picked on. We all know what children can be and how they pick on those who are not coping. Sometimes children need to have an 'out' group in order to feel at one with the 'in' group, unfortunately. Children may be ostracized for all sorts of reasons – because it's not cool to be shy and polite, or clever, or wear glasses, or not have a Swatch watch – or have a learning disability. At our school, our first task is to build up their self-confidence. Once they are happy in their environment it all flows from there.

Bullying

Bullying is one major reason why parents might consider removing their dyspraxic child from mainstream school. Although all schools now have to have anti-bullying policies in place, it is clearly a huge problem for many youngsters, even those without learning disabilities. Bullying is the reason behind 18 per cent of the 112,825 calls Childline receives every year. A 2003 survey by the Thomas Coram Research Unit found that more than half of all primary and secondary school pupils felt that bullying was 'a big problem' or 'quite a problem' in their school. The survey looked at Year 5 and Year 8 pupils and found that just over a half (51 per cent) of the younger pupils had been bullied during the term, compared with 28 per cent of the older ones. About 60 per cent of the children felt that their schools dealt effectively with bullying, but many felt that adults – parents and teachers – were still inclined not to take it seriously, nor to listen to their concerns. Many also felt that reporting the bullying to staff or parents was likely to result in reprisals from the bullies, either in school or outside school hours.

Childline's conference on bullying in March 2003 set out some helpful strategies such as 'mentoring' and 'buddying' for children who have been bullied. Childline has also started the CHIPS initiative (Childline in Partnership with Schools) which supports schools in setting up schemes run by and for children and young people. Researchers have found that, not surprisingly, children with poor social skills and low self-esteem were more likely to be the victims of a 'vicious cycle' of bullying.

The National Pyramid Trust is an organization dedicated to improving the self-confidence and self-esteem of primary school children, usually around Year 3. The Trust works with schools, statutory and voluntary agencies to set up local Pyramid Clubs. All the children in one school year have their emotional and social needs assessed and those who seem to need special help and a boost to their confidence are invited to join a ten-week, activity-based Pyramid Club where they can have fun, make friends and develop self-esteem and social skills. The Trust also has a leaflet for parents on 'Building your Child's Self-Esteem'. Although not specifically aimed at children with developmental problems like dyspraxia, it could benefit them. Contact details on p. 92.

Learning aids

Sometimes, small changes to the way a subject is taught can make all the difference. A sloping board may be easier for children to write on than a flat desk. The Dyscovery Centre in Cardiff (contact details on p. 89) sells a variety of aids specially designed for dyspraxic children, including angled writing boards, seat wedges, pencil grips and special 'training' scissors. It's suggested that dyspraxic children pay special attention to posture, too – sitting straight on a chair with their feet flat on the ground and sitting somewhere they don't have to twist round to look at the teacher. It's very easy for a child whose co-ordination is poor, and who is concentrating hard on her handwriting, to slip and fall off her chair. Many Local Education Authorities have Outreach Workers with special expertise in special-needs teaching who can offer all sorts of practical hints and tips on how to make learning easier for dyspraxic children.

5

Dyspraxia and the Teenage Years

Adolescence is a time of change – physical, emotional and practical. It's often a time of turmoil as well, with young people seeming like near-adults at one moment and little children the next. It can be perplexing and infuriating for everyone, including them! Having a disability of any kind can just make these years that bit more difficult, both for the youngster with dyspraxia and for her family. Parents want to encourage their children to become as independent as possible, help them to face the future with confidence and not over-protect them. There are bound to be additional concerns for a child with a developmental disorder.

Changing schools

The first big change that children have to face is the transition from primary to secondary school. This incorporates several changes at once – moving from a familiar environment, perhaps within walking distance of home, to a large school campus which may be miles away. Travelling to school is often the first hurdle. Then, instead of being taught by one, familiar teacher in the same classroom all the time, a child has to find her way to different classrooms for each lesson period, and will be taught by a whole series of new teachers. She may have left some, or all, of her friends and have to make new ones. She will be expected to take more responsibility for herself – turning up with sports kit, cookery equipment or whatever on the right day, taking down details of homework in different subjects, getting the work done, handing it in to the right person at the right time. It's not always an easy transition for even the best-organized child. For someone with dyspraxia, it will present additional challenges.

How can parents help? First, by liaising with the school well in advance, so that both the child and everyone who is likely to come into contact with her knows what to expect and what difficulties she is likely to face. Experts recommend several visits to the school

35

campus, so that the child can begin to familiarize herself with the layout. As well as helping her, it will boost her confidence if she can actually help some of the other newcomers to find their way about.

Has the school had other dyspraxic pupils? What sort of help were they able to offer? For instance, if a child has problems copying down notes, perhaps a helper could do this for him, or he could be allowed to use a small tape-recorder or Dictaphone. Computer keyboards are an alternative for those with handwriting problems. Tasks can be broken down into small, manageable chunks with aids to memory like diaries and Post-It notes. Simple strategies like colour-coding the child's timetable and exercise books, notes and files can be really useful in helping him to remember that green means English, blue means maths, red means science. Talk to the PE staff if the child is very slow at dressing and undressing, so that extra time can be allowed. Communication is the key. By the time a child is old enough for secondary school his parents may well have devised all kinds of 'coping strategies' which can be passed on to his teachers and other helpers. Many of the Dyspraxia Foundation's local groups have information about these. For instance, to avoid panic and confusion on school mornings, lay out the child's clothes the night before in the order he will need to put them on – e.g. undies on top! The same applies to school bags and games kit. Zips and Velcro fastenings are often easier to cope with than fiddly buttons.

Ideally, of course, you should find out what the school's policy is on inclusion before you decide this is the right school for your child – although, in some areas, parents don't always get a place at their first choice of school. It helps, too, if your child goes to the same school as one or more of his primary-school friends, or if the new school can provide a 'buddy' to help him through any initial difficulties.

Janet feels that the fact that her daughter Eleanor was diagnosed in primary school and given a lot of support has helped her make the transition to high school.

Aids like writing slopes and laptops can help keep children in mainstream school. I made a point of telling all Ellie's primary teachers about her dyspraxia, every year, and they all did their best to help her. Now she's 12, I still do things for her that mums would expect to do for a younger child. She has a transparent pencil case so she knows just what is in it and I make sure her school bag is packed the night before. I also had a card printed for her, with her name and ten basic tasks she has problems with, like finding her way around and keeping up with written work, so that if she gets lost she can hand the card to any member of staff. That seems to have given her confidence in a huge new school!

She does have learning support in the shape of a laptop, and help with her cookery and science lessons. In the laboratory they have found her a stool with a back to it, unlike the three-legged stools the other children use. She likes art and history and classical studies, enjoys practical work, and is keen to learn.

She has two really good friends but, on the whole, has always found it hard to make and keep friends. At primary school her peers found her babyish and I was forever picking up the pieces of broken friendships.

I have mixed feelings about inclusion. Ellie would get extra attention and the chance to shine in a special school, but at the high school she is gaining life skills. Her dad and I have always encouraged her and told her she can do anything she sets her mind to.

Parents report very different levels of support for dyspraxic children in secondary schools. One mum was brushed off with a 'we teach all children in the same way in this school.' Another had her 13-year-old daughter come home in tears because she had had to run round the playing-field on her own as it took her so long to get into her games kit. One lad was accused of 'attention-seeking', and the brother of one dyspraxic boy was asked, 'Aren't you ashamed to have a brother like J?' There is sometimes a tendency for the child to hide his problems beneath a veneer of being 'the clown of the class'.

Adults with dyspraxia often look back on their schooldays with some bitterness, with PE lessons being a particularly traumatic experience for many – even those who, like Alex, had actually been diagnosed with dyspraxia.

'I cannot express how hateful they were,' says Alex, who is now 21.

In academic subjects, if someone is not very good they are put in a lower set with others of similar ability. At my school, dyspraxics like me were made to compete with the best athletes in the class. It was unbearably humiliating and made me so unhappy when everyone was watching me panting in last – every single time – in cross-country running, or I could not manage to hit the ball a single time in tennis. No other subject treats students like this. It is cruel. No wonder we have a problem with obesity and children not exercising in this country. The Government should implement a sets-based system, as it does in other subjects.

The PE teachers I had were all either cruel or patronizing and had no idea what to do if someone was struggling with their subject.

Adolescence is a sensitive time, and teenagers who sometimes feel embarrassed to leave the house at all do not need to be dressed in ludicrous outfits and made to humiliate themselves in front of their peer group.

Eleven-year-old Louise is allowed 30 hours of one-to-one help in her new school.

'It has changed from primary school,' comments Janey, her mother.

Her helper does guide her, but also knows when to stand back and let Lou have that bit more independence. A lot does depend on the child's personality. Lou is jovial and funny and everyone likes her. She is also a big girl for her age which makes her less likely to be bullied. She is getting all the help she needs but I do hear about other families having a tough time.

Cheryl says that she and her 15-year-old son Ben are 'muddling through'. His school has been reasonably supportive – certainly on the academic side – but is poor at dealing with bullying.

We have found ways of dealing with Ben's problems as they arose. For instance, he has two files for homework. The red file is 'to be done' and the green file is 'done'. He has a school–home diary which his teachers check, and he doesn't go out of the door without my asking him if he has his money, his lunch, his phone and his keys! In some ways he is old for his age – he's over six feet tall and shaving – in other ways, worryingly young. For example, he has little road sense and is very poor at judging time, speed and distance, especially if he is trying to hold a conversation at the same time. Games lessons are still a problem. He will never be a footballer, but luckily friends seem to have taken him under their wing and introduced him to different sports like golf, hockey and trampolining, which he enjoys. He's studying languages, IT, media studies and science for GCSEs and the school has arranged extra lessons with a special needs group, going over subjects he finds especially difficult.

For some children, special education will still be the preferred option, as Catherine Allen of the Home School in north London explains.

Children come here suffering from clinical depression and later get their GCSEs and are able to face the world with confidence. It just isn't true that all children do better in mainstream education. In a large secondary school, an average teacher will see perhaps 200 children every week. It can be very difficult to remember that little Johnny has co-ordination problems. The education our children get here is not very different, but because we are a small group we can teach to the child's own strengths. Everyone thinks in a different way, and we can work out how each child learns and how to present information to that child individually. This just isn't possible in a huge school environment.

Our children are able to spend some time on sport, doing things like riding bikes and rowing that improve co-ordination. We also do art work that will improve their fine and gross motor skills – not just painting and drawing but also collage and 3D modelling in clay. We offer extra handwriting lessons too. Although word-processing skills are taught as well, at the end of the day you need handwriting too.

Children come to us at 11 and stay to 16 or 17. After that some go on to study for academic qualifications and some learn vocational skills. Building up their confidence and self-esteem is a vital part of what we do.

By the time children reach secondary-school age, you can't drag them to school and if they are not coping or are being bullied, they will just leg it!

Will the child grow out of it?

There isn't yet a huge body of research into what happens to dyspraxic children as they grow up. Parents often ask if the child will grow out of his or her difficulties, and the answer has to be that we just don't know. There are, as yet, only about half-a-dozen studies looking at teenagers with dyspraxia and the picture they give is mixed. A piece of research from Australia in the 1980s suggested that many less severely affected children would grow out of the problem; another, from Sweden, found that problems were more persistent in children whose dyspraxia was combined with another condition such as ADHD. Finnish studies came to the conclusion that by the age of about 17, half of dyspraxic children seemed to have grown out of their dyspraxia.

Psychologist Margaret Cousins of Lancaster University is conducting an ongoing study of what happens as dyspraxic children grow up. She has found that early intervention in childhood makes a big difference – not least, to the child's self-confidence – and that, as children mature, it helps if therapy is targeted on individual difficulties.

Obviously, things do change as children grow up. Some skills become less important, others more so. Older students can make choices about what subjects they study and can give up those they dislike most. Given the right kind of teaching, with additional support if necessary, young people with dyspraxia can and do get GCSEs and A levels, NVQs and university degrees. Ms Cousins also suggests concentrating on the things a child is interested in and/or good at. People with dyspraxia have been known to shine at art, football, tennis or playing musical instruments. Gyms and sports centres offer teenagers the opportunity to enjoy physical activities suited to their needs. A young person who can't cope with team games might still enjoy swimming, riding, jogging or trampolining.

Teenage traumas

Growing up is not just about educational achievement, though. Children with developmental disorders have to face all the usual teenage traumas – family and relationship problems, career choices and so on. Parents want to help, but don't always know what help to offer. Tears, moods and sulks are commonplace. As one parent put it, 'I'm never sure if it's her dyspraxia that's the problem or her hormones!'

'People tend to be less patient with teenagers who keep losing things or can't find their way about, than they are with younger children,' comments Fiona, mother of 13-year-old Kerry.

> Teens with dyspraxia tend to be outsiders as they're not in with the football or netball crowd. Kerry is quite young for her age and not very interested in boyfriends yet, but older girls I've known have missed out on dates because they tend to be rather overweight and have poor posture, which is a big issue for girls. I think teenage problems are magnified in dyspraxic kids. Boys tend to take it out on other people, becoming delinquent, and girls are more likely to self-harm.
>
> I've always tried to be open and honest with my daughter. We sit down and talk about things like drug problems, other people's attitudes, and bullying. TV soaps can be a good starting-point. We talk through the storylines as we do the ironing!
>
> Personal hygiene is occasionally a problem for young teens with memory problems, because they can't remember when they last had a shower or when it's hair-wash day. Kerry coped well with her first period as we had practised beforehand and she was well prepared.

Mums with teenage daughters say that practising using sanitary protection in advance helps their daughters to deal with menstruation. Some girls still find it upsetting or embarrassing, but no more so than their non-dyspraxic sisters. For girls with co-ordination problems, it's especially important to experiment with different types of towel, with and without 'wings', to find a type that suits them best. Girls will need to be shown exactly where and how to stick them to their knickers. Some young teenagers worry a lot about possible 'leaks' and need plenty of reassurance. Carrying spare supplies and an extra pair of pants in the school bag can help girls to feel secure.

Dr Amanda Kirby of the Dyscovery Centre in Cardiff has written a book about teenagers and dyspraxia. She says that it's important for parents to balance their natural feelings of protectiveness with the need to help young people develop appropriate skills for independent living. She reminds parents to look at their teenager as someone with a different style of learning, rather than someone who is 'difficult'.

> With plenty of support and good organizational strategies, they will be able to make progress towards independent living slowly, but steadily. They need to be encouraged to do things for themselves, like all adolescents – ranging from making a snack in the kitchen and clearing up after themselves, to catching the right bus to visit a friend, or doing some simple shopping. Mastering these skills can take time so parents have to be patient.

Dr Kirby reminds parents about the things that are important to all teenagers – the way they look, the way they relate to others, sporting prowess in the case of boys – and some girls! Teens with dyspraxia don't have to miss out. If your teenage son isn't good at football, he may enjoy and stand out at some other kind of physical activity – swimming, canoeing, trampolining, golf or horse-riding, for instance. Or he may enjoy completely different hobbies like pottery, photography, computer games or taking care of animals.

> It can be easier to get away with being a non-sporty girl, so in that sense it may be harder for boys to fit in with their peer group. Teenage boys with dyspraxia may be good at showing their 'feminine' side by being caring – which is great for Mum but not for their peers.
> Don't underestimate the importance of looks and clothes, either. With many teenagers, having the right gear is the first step to street cred. Let them go shopping with their friends or maybe an older sibling so that they can be aware of, and enjoy, trying out young fashion. Otherwise there's a risk that they will end up looking like their parents and that makes it harder for them to fit in.

In her researches Dr Kirby has found that relationships tend to happen later for young people with dyspraxia.

'They may be emotionally immature. At 14 or 15 they are still sorting themselves out and tend not to be ready for relationships,' she comments. 'Secure friendships are very important to these young people as they may have been bullied. Again, confidence and self-esteem is the key and anything parents, siblings and teachers can do to build this up is helpful.'

Becoming independent

As Dr Kirby says, it's never too early to begin helping your teenager in the quest for independence. Eventually he will have to choose a career and probably plan for some kind of higher education. Going to university will involve living away from home so the more everyday 'life skills' he has acquired, the better. An organization called SKILL (contact details on p. 92) can give information about further and higher education and employment opportunities for people with disabilities. This includes information about financial assistance in the form of Disabled Students' Allowances, and about employing support workers. They also publish books about particular professions and their suitability for disabled workers, including case histories of those who have entered the profession. If your teenager is interested in working in architecture, art, the law, science and engineering, he can obtain these books at a special price.

Colleges and universities can be very sympathetic and helpful in meeting the needs of students with disabilities, including dyspraxia. Recent research by educational psychologist Madeleine Portwood into dyspraxia awareness at further educational institutions found that most responded positively. Brunel and Birmingham Universities came top of the list. Only 4 per cent of the colleges who responded to the survey reported no policy, support or special arrangements for students with dyspraxia.

If a young person wants to leave school to go on to college, university or work-based training and has a statement of special needs, the Connexions service (formerly the Careers Service, but with a wider remit) will do another assessment to work out what special help he or she will need. The Connexions service can also help non-statemented young people with special needs to make the transition to adult life. (Contact details for Connexions Direct on p. 91 or see your local phone book.)

Adults with dyspraxia interviewed for this book said that college and university days were much less stressful for them than their schooldays, with the college authorities doing what they could to help, even though most of them had not been given an official diagnosis. Study skills learned at school can be adapted for university, with extra time given for exams and more use of word-processors and/or access to other students or staff lecture notes, if taking notes is a problem. Universities all have Disability Advisers or Co-Ordinators to help organize such concessions. SKILL can give you information about these.

Throughout the teenage years it's more important than ever to think positively. As one parent wrote to the Dyspraxia Foundation's Newsletter,

> When our son was diagnosed, aged 5, we were given a great list of things he would find difficult, or would not achieve . . . he worked hard at every task he was set and after five years of therapy, he had improved in leaps and bounds.
>
> Last summer, he completed three years at college and qualified as a chef. He has achieved everything he ever wanted . . . and is no different from any other 19-year-old. With love, encouragement and willpower, children with dyspraxia can achieve anything they want to!

6
Dyspraxia in Adult Life

Experts agree that the sooner a child is diagnosed with this condition, the better. Not only does a diagnosis enable parents to start looking for sources of help – physiotherapy, occupational therapy, extra support at school – but it also enables everyone around the dyspraxic child to make allowances. Once everyone, from parents and siblings to teachers, understands what is really happening, they can help the child to develop coping strategies which will lead to increased self-confidence and higher self-esteem. The social cost of ignoring dyspraxia, or assuming that children with the condition will grow out of it, can be high. One long-term study found that as many as 80 per cent of the children diagnosed at 7 were, by the age of 22, unemployed, had broken the law, were alcohol or drug misusers or had mental health problems.

Living with dyspraxia

Sadly, many current treatment options were simply not available for the generation who are now adults living with dyspraxia.

'Adults do get left out,' says Elizabeth, who wasn't diagnosed until she was in her late thirties.

> There is an assumption that we grow out of it, although in my opinion some of us just develop better coping strategies. Some people's co-ordination does improve as they get older. Mine didn't. Even if it does, many people are left with a poor short-term memory and bad organizational skills which can lead to difficulties and misunderstandings in the workplace.

These are the people who *were* stigmatized as clumsy, lazy, stupid or just a bit strange. Many GPs still know little about the condition, and as one adult with dyspraxia said, 'You might not approach your GP anyway, just to tell him that you had a terrible sense of direction, couldn't drive, or had problems using a tin-opener!'

Many adults with dyspraxia have had very mixed experiences with health professionals over the years.

'The first doctor my mother took me to said confidently that she should send me to a special school and that I would never learn to read and write,' says Alex, 21.

> I now have a degree in English Literature so I think it's safe to say we have proved him wrong.
>
> After that my mother took me to another specialist who was very good. I had physiotherapy throughout infant school and was encouraged to do things like learn to swim and ride a bike, as well as playing musical instruments. Although I never developed any level of proficiency, at least I learned that I could do things if I tried.

It's very easy for people who have grown up with low self-esteem, feeling stupid and useless and wondering why they are not like other people, to develop mental health problems like anxiety or depression, or turn to alcohol or drugs. Many, like Alex, have gone on to prove their ill-informed teachers wrong, but they admit that it has been a struggle.

Take Breda, for instance. At 45, Breda has no fewer than two MSc degrees and is a member of MENSA, the organization for those whose IQ places them in the top 2 per cent of the population. She also has dyspraxia, which means that she can't drive a car and gets lost if she leaves the main street of her home town. She has handwriting problems, is extremely disorganized, has no sense of direction and is a very poor judge of speed, time and distance.

> I was always told I was lazy and stupid and at school I just assumed that everyone else was cleverer than me. I was always one of the last to finish when copying from the blackboard and didn't do well in exams.
>
> I found it hard to follow the rules in school, because I didn't really understand them. Corporal punishment was used in my primary school and I was actually afraid of many of my teachers. I didn't understand why I was being punished – I honestly never meant to be troublesome. I thought it was my fault, that if I just tried harder things would work out for me. Growing up with

undiagnosed dyspraxia was awful. I loved my parents but I couldn't understand why they had inflicted life on me.

Breda struggled at her grammar school but eventually managed to study maths and physics at A level and went on to university where she took a BSc and then two higher degrees.

It's unfortunate that I was not assessed and diagnosed as a child, so that I would have had a chance of managing my condition better, and discovering more of my strengths. I still think I am luckier than most in that I did eventually get to discover what I was good at. Many dyspraxics don't. They struggle all their lives with basic, simple tasks and don't get a chance to find out what amazing talents they may have in other areas.

Support for adults

The Dyspraxia Foundation has an adult support group and can also provide leaflets about the condition which will help employers to understand the difficulties faced by people with dyspraxia in their working environment. The Disability Rights Commission (contact details on p. 94) can offer advice in cases of discrimination and unfair dismissal. Their website is a good source of information on employer and employee rights and responsibilities.

Under the terms of the Disability Discrimination Act 1995, an employer is obliged to make 'reasonable adjustments' to accommo-date the needs of disabled employees. The Act originally applied only to firms employing more than 15 people, but from now applies to all employers. The Act covers those people whose ability to carry out day-to-day activities is affected by a physical or mental impairment on a long-term basis. This can, of course, include people with dyspraxia, but the issue is not clear-cut because the degree of impairment caused varies from person to person and also depends on your job and working environment. If you are in the right job and the right environment and you are only mildly affected you may not need any extra help from your employer.

Employers must not, by law, treat those with disabilities less favourably with regard to promotion, training, receiving extra benefits, or dismissal.

Because dyspraxia is a *hidden* disability which may not be immediately obvious, some employers will not know how the working environment can be adapted for someone with the condition. It's also the case that dyspraxia affects working people in different ways, so it is often up to the employee to explain exactly what he can do and what he finds most difficult. The Disability Rights Commission explains that 'adjustments' can cover things like flexible working hours, special training, buying extra equipment or even employing an assistant to help the disabled person carry out their job most effectively. The Disability Employment Adviser at your local JobCentre (contact details in phone book) will be able to help you both, including giving you information about the Access to Work scheme, which can sometimes help to fund special equipment for those with impairments. There is also an organization called the Employers' Forum on Disability (contact details on p. 94) which can help and advise employers on best practice. Like all employees with disabilities, those with dyspraxia are keen to point out that there are *advantages* to employing them – like low rates of absenteeism and, in the case of dyspraxics, an ability to 'think outside the box' and bring a fresh approach to many work issues.

In spite of attempts to integrate people with all kinds of disabilities into normal working life, discrimination does still happen, as many adults with dyspraxia are finding to their cost.

Martin, for example, was dismissed from his office job and is currently taking his previous employer to an Industrial Tribunal. He felt that his employer never really recognized dyspraxia as a disability.

'My line manager said that I was disorganized,' says Martin, who has an HND and post-graduate qualifications.

> In a sense, being highly qualified worked against me, because my employer claimed that if I could study at a further education college, my disability couldn't be that bad. What they never understood was that special arrangements were made for me at college. I was given extra time for exams and allowed to use a word-processor because my fine motor skills and handwriting were poor.
> At work I was eventually seen by an occupational psychologist, who said that if my work was re-organized and broken up into

small, manageable tasks, I could cope perfectly well. However the list of recommendations he made was seen by the company as a burden and implemented only half-heartedly. The human resources department even said they were prepared to adjust my workload, but only for three months, even though I tried to explain to them that I had a disability which wasn't going to go away.

Another problem was that the courts wouldn't accept that I was dyspraxic, because the diagnosis had been made by an educational psychologist when I was a child and confirmed by an occupational psychologist more recently, rather than a doctor! I would definitely like to see more awareness of the condition among employers.

Martin currently has another job, as a support worker for people with physical and learning disabilities.

'I originally started as a temp and was asked to join the team on a permanent basis. I do feel that employers should use our gifts and make the most of them,' he says.

Not all employers are so unsympathetic. Kate, like Martin, is highly qualified and, at 31, is currently combining her PhD studies with part-time tutoring of special-needs children at a private school. She was only diagnosed with dyspraxia three years ago.

I did have a full-time teaching job at another school which threw me totally, and eventually I had a nervous breakdown. Looking back, a busy school environment where I had to deal with thirty children at once was totally the wrong place for me! Luckily, there was a school counsellor who knew about dyspraxia.

The Head at my present school, where I teach small groups of children with learning difficulties, has a disability herself and she has been really sympathetic. I am allowed the concessions I need. I don't have to go to staff meetings because there is too much sensory overload for me and I don't know which notes to take. I have help with writing reports. I don't have to do lunch duties, and as my physical co-ordination is poor I don't have to help with stacking chairs or anything like that.

Over the years Kate has learned that admitting she has a disability and asking for help when she needs it often produces a sympathetic response.

I am really hopeless at tasks which seem simple to other people, like using a stapler or photocopier, so I just ask for help with them. I go to a local gym which I enjoy. I can't set the machines but the instructors are happy to help me out. I use a treadmill for running and also do special exercises to strengthen my back and improve my co-ordination. I think you have to accept that there are certain things you just can't do – I will never be any good at driving or doing keep fit – but being a gym member has improved my posture and toned me up. I took in leaflets about dyspraxia to show the instructors and they were more than willing to learn and be educated about it. I think that if society was more accepting and understanding of those of us who are different, dyspraxia would not be a disability!

Choosing a career

The Dyspraxia Foundation points out that there are ways round most of the problems faced by employees with dyspraxia. They are often creative and original thinkers, so, in the right job, can be an asset to any organization. However, even more than everyone else, they need careful guidance when it comes to choosing an appropriate career. The Foundation suggests that anyone contemplating career choices – or a career move in later life – should make a list of their strengths and weaknesses and try to find something that fits in with them.

Above all, you should choose a job you are going to enjoy. Remember that many skills and talents are not measurable by exam results. You could be a persuasive talker who would do well in some sort of sales career, or the sort of gentle soul who is brilliant at 'empathizing' with troubled children, adults or confused elderly people. You should also make a point of:

- **reading** as much as you can about jobs and careers and the qualifications required – your local library and the Internet are good sources of information. Publishers Kogan Page publish a whole series of careers books you might find useful;

50

- **consulting** all the people who can help you to make your choice. That could include parents and family, teachers at school, Special-Needs Careers Advisers at the local Careers Service (Connexions), or the Disability Service Team at the JobCentre. Listen carefully to what they say but remember that ultimately it is your life and your decision;
- **studying** for a further qualification if that's what is needed to take you nearer to your ultimate goal;
- **adapting** your future career to take account of your special difficulties, whether those involve physical co-ordination, short-term memory problems or lack of organizational skills. You have probably learned 'ways round the problem' at school which can easily be taken forward into the world of work – for instance, using lots of memory aids like diaries, timetables and Post-It notes.

As with any career choice, you need to strike a balance between aiming high – if you don't try for the job you really want, you will never know whether you could have made it or not – and being realistic about your talents and abilities, as well as your disability. If you faint at the sight of blood, a career as a surgeon is not for you; if you're shy and a bit of a loner, you will not shine as a holiday rep – but that all applies to job-hunters who don't have dyspraxia too.

Job hunting

Similarly, the advice the Foundation gives to members about applying for jobs and attending interviews could equally well apply to candidates without a disability. It's always an idea to fill out application forms in pencil first (or take a copy and work on that) so that it doesn't matter if you make a mistake. Some organizations encourage candidates to download application forms from their websites, fill them in on the computer screen and email them back, which is great for those whose IT skills are better than their handwriting.

You could try asking someone to give you a 'mock' interview to see how you get on. It always helps to find out about the company you will (hopefully) be working for so that you have questions to ask which don't concern salary and holidays! You could always ask what a typical working day will be like if you are stumped for an appropriate question. That is also a good way of finding out if there are parts of the job you will find especially challenging.

Although you need to look smart, it makes sense to wear clothes you feel comfortable in. Allow more time than you think you could possibly need to get to the interview, so that you don't panic if the train or bus is late. Always write down the instructions for getting to the interview, the name of the person you need to ask for, and the telephone number, in case you are unavoidably delayed. A trial run is a good idea as well.

What should you tell your employer about your dyspraxia?

If you are only mildly affected by the condition and you are sure that it will not affect your ability to do the job at all, you're not obliged to say anything. So much depends on the degree of disability, and on the job. Will you be working as part of a team, in a busy office with a lot happening all around you, or will you be left to get on with the job in your own time and at your own pace? Which would suit you better?

It's quite likely that if you mention 'dyspraxia' to a boss or potential boss you will be greeted with a blank look. Taking along some of the Dyspraxia Foundation's literature will be very useful. If you know your dyspraxia means you have poor organizational skills and a poor short-term memory, you should be able to show your employer how you manage these difficulties, with the aid of flow-charts, 'To Do' lists, colour-coded files and so on. It is quite likely that you won't know if there are parts of the job you can't cope with until you are asked to do them, so be prepared for that. Remember, you wouldn't have been invited for an interview if the person on the other side of the desk had not thought you had skills and talents to offer. Dyspraxia is not the whole story! Always be positive and emphasize all the things you are good at.

The Disability Rights Commission points out that while you are under no legal obligation to declare your disability at the interview, doing so will alert your employer and make it easy to talk about, and work out 'reasonable adjustments' at this early stage. Otherwise, if you later make a claim for discrimination, your employer can counter-claim that he did not know you had a disability when he took you on. They also advise that if your special needs are not met, you should ask for a meeting as soon as possible to discuss the issue, and take proper notes at the meeting in case you need to make a claim under the Act.

Strategies you have already used at school and college can be adapted in the workplace. Make a point of writing down, or typing out, any instructions you are given. Instructions for the use of office equipment, from the photocopier to the coffee machine, will benefit all employees. If you use a computer, make sure you are sitting comfortably. Spell-checkers are useful, as are keyboard shortcuts for those who find a mouse hard to use. If you work better in a quiet atmosphere with few distractions, see if you can arrange to have your desk partitioned off, or even an office on your own.

Flexitime is often beneficial as it enables workers with dyspraxia to start the day in an orderly manner, perhaps prioritizing tasks for the day and breaking them up into small, achievable chunks on the 'To Do' list before the rest of the team get in and the phones start ringing. You might even be allowed to play soothing music through headphones if you find you lose concentration when there's too much going on around you. There is usually something that can be done to enable you to do the job, as long as your employer and fellow-workers have the right attitude. Companies whose human resources departments are flexible and imaginative can also find ways to make use of the creative talents of those with conditions like dyspraxia.

'We are "extreme machines",' says Breda, 'brilliant at some things and truly awful at others. Large organizations, who are always saying they need abstract thinkers and those with the ability to look at issues in a different way, should be taking advantage of that.'

Claiming benefits

Those who are severely affected by dyspraxia and those who have additional problems like dyslexia may not be able to cope with a full-time job. Like everyone else with a disability, you may be entitled to benefits like Disability Living Allowance or Incapacity Benefit if you are in this position. As is often the case with the benefits system, however, this is not a clearcut issue.

'We have tried to produce information sheets on eligibility for benefits,' says a spokesperson from Nottingham-based support group Dyspraxia Connexion.

> However, we have always found it impossible, because it depends so much on each individual case. If we say, 'Those who have dyspraxia are entitled to this or that benefit,' it is not necessarily true. Eligibility for benefit depends – understandably, and quite rightly – on individual needs. The problem is in defining the degree of disability, not the dyspraxia label. There is a big discrepancy between those who are only mildly affected, who can cope with the right job, if their employer is supportive, and those who are more severely affected who find it impossible to hold down a full-time job at all.
>
> We are aware of adults who are in supported employment who are eligible for Disability Living Allowance and Incapacity Benefit, others who feel under pressure to earn a living and prefer part-time work, and some who can't work at all.
>
> We are available to help people fill out the forms for Disability Living Allowance and make sure the answers they give are accurate. There is a box which has to be filled in by a 'professional' like a doctor and we can tick that for them. In order to claim Incapacity Benefit, most people would need to see a doctor but the Benefits Agency can also contact other relevant professionals like educational or occupational psychologists.

If you want to know about more about benefits to which you might be entitled, a first step might be to call the Benefits Enquiry Line for those with disabilities (contact details on p. 93).

Coping with everyday life

Coping with dyspraxia in adult life isn't just about work, of course. Co-ordination difficulties affect adults differently and, depending on their severity, can make the simplest task seem daunting. Preparing meals and cleaning up afterwards can take twice as long, since those with dyspraxia find cutting, peeling, stirring, mixing, opening cans, unscrewing jars, and pouring liquid into a cup or container hard to master, and spills are common. Even dressing can be difficult, with some dyspraxics resorting to tearing their clothes on and off, or living in easy-to-manage loose T-shirts and pull-on trousers or skirts.

Elizabeth says that until she was diagnosed in her late thirties, she had no idea why she found the 'business' of living, including everyday tasks like cooking, driving or even bathing the baby, such a struggle.

I am dyslexic as well. Many dyspraxics have other conditions which complicate their lives. My doctor was not helpful and it was only by chance that I was eventually diagnosed. I just happened to have a friend who was a paediatric physiotherapist who suggested I might be dyspraxic.

I found that nothing came naturally to me. Even things like cooking and ironing had to be broken down into small steps for me to follow, and even then it was a tremendous effort. I have had the help of two very good occupational therapists who have showed me how to organize my life better. They told me to write down everything I have to do in a book, which is something I still do. I would like to see much more awareness of dyspraxia in the NHS, with the same sort of help available for us as there is for people recovering after stroke illness, as we share many of their problems.

Driving

Driving is a big issue for people with dyspraxia. Some do master it, but the reaction of most of those interviewed for this book was 'I would be lethal on the roads!' The Dyspraxia Foundation has a leaflet on the subject which explains that the required co-ordination – needing to steer, concentrate, tell left from right, use hands and feet together on different tasks, judge speed and distance *and* be aware of what is happening among other road users – is a daunting prospect. Of course, it is sometimes possible to manage without a car, depending on your work and social commitments and where you live, but obtaining a licence is certainly useful. Fortunately, the Department of Transport has a Mobility Advice and Information Service (MAVIS) (contact details on p. 93). They run special Assessment Centres around the country where disabled drivers can be advised in a safe and understanding environment. The Driving Standards Agency (contact details on p. 94) also has a special needs team who can give advice to potential drivers with disabilities. Since 2000, the Driving Theory Test has been conducted as a touch-screen, computer-based test which is designed to be user-friendly for all candidates. There is a practice session lasting up to 15 minutes to allow candidates to become familiar with the system.

Some driving schools have special courses for those with disabilities. BSM, for example, runs BSM Mobility Training, which was set up in 1994 to meet the needs of older and less able drivers. BSM Instructors are trained at the Queen Elizabeth Foundation Mobility Training Centre in Surrey, to ensure that drivers with disabilities get the support and flexibility they need to develop skills behind the wheel.

'Staff will advise on arranging an assessment of fitness to drive and planning lessons,' says their spokesperson.

Each student receives an individually tailored tuition plan incorporating practical training and assistance with the theory test. We operate automatic dual-control Vauxhall Corsas with power-assisted steering and seat-height adjusters. Cars have specialist adaptations for a variety of disabilities, including accelerator pedals which can be used by the left or right foot, push–pull levers for brake, accelerator and indicators, and a 6-way infra-red unit to operate other controls. Staff can also advise on choosing a car and on the Motability scheme for disabled drivers.

If you plan to take lessons, find out whether there are any local driving instructors who have taught anyone with special needs. The Foundation can also give you tips and hints about how to pass your test and cope with driving. They recommend learning in an automatic car as you have less to think about, and marking the right-hand side of the steering wheel with a sticker so that it's easier to remember which side is which.

It could happen, of course, that driving is really not for you; if that's the case you will find out during your lessons. Try not to be too discouraged. Instead, remind yourself of the money you will save by taking buses and taxis instead!

If you need help with practical tasks around the home you might find disability aids useful – these are available to help with anything from unscrewing jam jars to putting on your socks or stockings. Contact the Disabled Living Foundation (details on p. 94) and companies like Keep Able and Ways and Means (see pp. 94–5) for information.

Relationships are sometimes more complicated if you have a developmental disorder. Martin, who was diagnosed at 5, says he has always been something of a loner and had few friends as a child. Now in his mid-thirties, he is single and has had problems relating to women.

'I was once accused of sexual harassment and it was a sincere misunderstanding,' he says.

> A friend did tell me that I have a tendency to stand too close to people, which feels like invading their personal space, so I am more aware of it now. But I do feel it's a mistake to blame all one's personal failings on dyspraxia.

Kate says that she thinks the condition can cause more problems for men than for women.

'I always had lots of friends and a supportive family,' she says.

> I was always physically clumsy and couldn't do anything practical but it didn't affect my ability to form relationships with men. They seemed to like driving me about and opening wine bottles for me. These were things I couldn't do myself and it gave them a chance to show off and be macho. It must be harder if you are a man and you can't do these things.

Kay, who was diagnosed in her thirties, says that she had one very difficult relationship with a controlling boyfriend who used her condition as an excuse to 'take over'.

'Luckily I got out in time,' she says, 'and my current partner is a very gentle, caring person who is happy to let me do things in my own way and my own time.'

7

Who Can Help?

Because comparatively little is known about the causes of dyspraxia and there's not much research into the condition, there is no 'treatment' as such. Sadly, there is as yet no handy drug which has been proved to help co-ordination. Learning to cope with dyspraxia is something of a hit-and-miss affair involving a multi-disciplinary approach from health professionals. As is common in the National Health Service, the amount of help available locally tends to depend on where you live, and is patchy at best.

Children are much better catered for than adults because they are involved in the educational system, where there is much more awareness of 'special needs'. Schools and nurseries all have their Special Needs Co-ordinator or SENCO whose job is to identify ways in which 'different' children can be helped.

Help from your GP

Within the health system, many GPs are poorly informed about the condition, especially the way it affects adults. The Adult Dyspraxia Support Group recently carried out a survey of all 532 Primary Care Groups in England and their equivalent in Wales, Scotland and Northern Ireland. Less than one-fifth of all PCGs (a total of 97) returned the questionnaires and only *two* gave a completely positive answer – Huddersfield and Grampian. In these areas, it seems that there are

- GPs who would diagnose dyspraxia in adults;
- specialists to whom they can be referred;
- physio, OT and speech therapy services available to them.

More than 57 per cent of those PCGs who responded did not provide any services, although 69 per cent knew something about dyspraxia. The Dyspraxia Foundation reports that a lot of GPs contact them for information about how they can help their patients.

Alan was diagnosed with 'Clumsy Child Syndrome' while still at primary school, though neither he nor his parents were ever told and he didn't learn he had dyspraxia till he was 29, three years ago.

My GP was reasonably helpful, though he hadn't heard of dyspraxia before. Checking my records, he came across the 'Clumsy Child Syndrome' diagnosis, and then undertook to look for treatment on my behalf. However, he concluded that NHS treatment was not available to anyone with dyspraxia who was over 16, and from there on, finding treatment has been up to me!

Even when a child is diagnosed, it is often a matter of luck whether he sees a paediatrician with an interest in learning disorders, or whether he is referred for help to a physiotherapist, occupational therapist or speech therapist. Waiting times to see these specialists vary around the country and Foundation members report lengthy waits and lengthy drives to the nearest suitable practitioner.

If help for children with dyspraxia on the NHS is, at best, patchy, facilities for adults are virtually non-existent. Ray, a member of the Foundation's Adult Support group, says that his extensive researches had come up with no medical doctor in the Western world who is a specialist in dyspraxia in adults.

'There are Institutes in Eastern Europe like the Peto Institute in Hungary who treat co-ordination problems, but they specialize in cerebral palsy,' he says. 'Sweden seems to be many years ahead of Britain. All children there are given very thorough developmental checks and the connections between developmental disorders are recognized. Britain is lagging behind.'

Mary Colley, the Co-Ordinator of the DF's adult support group, underlines how poor the service is for adults with dyspraxia when she says that typically, members of the group were diagnosed by chance, and only after many years of difficulty.

I was diagnosed by an educational psychologist at university, and you can sometimes see a clinical psychologist or a neurologist on the NHS. Generally the medical profession is more interested in treating acquired dyspraxia – for instance, in patients who have suffered a stroke. I did manage to see two excellent occupational therapists but I had to really fight for them, and it's the luck of the draw who you get! I have compiled a list of private practitioners who can help. Some people find counselling or something like Cognitive Behavioural Therapy helpful, but generally I'm afraid that adults with dyspraxia are pretty much ignored.

Naturally, the Dyspraxia Foundation feels that with more recognition and awareness of the condition, this state of affairs will not continue. At present, it seems that one of the best ways to find the help you need is to contact the Foundation itself.

Help from the Foundation

The Dyspraxia Foundation was set up as the Dyspraxia Trust in 1987 by two mothers who had met at Great Ormond Street Hospital for Sick Children. It is a registered charity which changed its name in 1996. (Contact details are on p. 88.) Its objects are

- to support individuals and families affected by dyspraxia;
- to promote better diagnostic and treatment facilities for those affected;
- to help health and education professionals to assist those with dyspraxia;
- to promote awareness and understanding.

The Foundation has 34 support groups around the country and publishes a twice-yearly newsletter and an annual report. Local groups offer the chance for parents to meet others, share experiences and lobby for better local facilities. They also fund-raise and organize all kinds of events from visits to Cadbury World to outdoor activity weekends for children and parents.

Experts do agree that targeted help is most beneficial for both children and adults. In other words, if the main problem is poor physical co-ordination, then a physiotherapist might be the best person to help. If it's difficulty in managing daily life – anything from remembering appointments to operating household gadgets – try to see an occupational therapist. Speech therapy benefits those – mostly children – whose speech is very unclear, and some form of counselling or psychotherapy might be best for someone with self-esteem issues, relationship problems or the depression which seems all too common in adult dyspraxics who have grown up without knowing what their problem really was.

What a physiotherapist can do

'Therapy should be fun!' says Michele Lee, a physio who has devised her own method of working with youngsters with dyspraxia, and now runs a private clinic in Buckinghamshire. She has written two books on dyspraxia and regularly publishes papers in medical journals. Physiotherapy can help children's co-ordination, muscle tone, core stability, hand–eye co-ordination, directional awareness, body perception, and short-term visual and verbal memory. Ultimately, the treatment should increase the child's self-confidence and self-esteem, so that he or she begins to feel successful.

Michele assesses her young patients individually and tailors her exercise programme accordingly. Parents are asked to fill in a detailed questionnaire so that she can work out which areas should be concentrated on.

'My system works in eight-week blocks,' she explains.

I see the child once a week for an hour and there are also 15–20 minutes of home exercises to do every day. The emphasis is on core stability, working on the shoulders and trunk. For the first four weeks, we concentrate on co-ordination, organization, memory and motor skills, and in the last four weeks on hand exercises and more motor skills.

After that I see the child less frequently, reviewing his progress all the time until he is just coming back for an annual check-up. However, these children will probably need help all through childhood, especially when it comes to events like changing schools, revising for exams and taking up new hobbies. Bullying may also be an issue so the increase in self-confidence which comes when tasks are successfully completed is an important part of the treatment. Liaison with the child's school is also very important and we send information to the school together with an advice leaflet for the child's class and PE teachers.

Physiotherapy sessions for children are designed to be enjoyable as well as useful. Children wear informal, casual clothes like shorts and T-shirts and, depending on their needs, may be asked to do all kinds of exercises, for instance:

- 'wheelbarrows' – walking on hands with feet held;
- bunny hops;
- lying prone on a scooter board and propelling it around with the arms;
- drawing shapes in the air;
- writing on a blackboard;
- playing constructional games like Lego;
- throwing and catching balls and bean-bags, either to himself or to someone else;
- playing skittles;
- throwing bean-bags into different-sized boxes;
- playing 'pick-up-sticks';
- playing 'Simon says' and touching parts of the body to order;
- practising following a sequence of instructions – for example, walking round in a circle, then giving two hops and two claps, in the right order.

There are lots and lots more simple games and exercises which children can benefit from, and enjoy, from the age of about 4 onwards, although Michele says she is happy to advise parents of even younger children.

Where adults are concerned, she points out that there is no research evidence to prove that physiotherapy benefits adults with dyspraxia.

'Adults I have spoken to seem to have more problems with organizational skills, and derive more benefit from occupational therapy,' she says.

However, it is important for adults with dyspraxia to maintain their general fitness levels and muscle strength, Fortunately, today's generation of 20- and 30-somethings – who may already have been treated in childhood – are aware of the need to keep fit. It's important to find an activity that you really enjoy. Long walks, at a good speed so that you maintain cardiovascular fitness, are good – or you could try badminton, horse-riding, fishing, golf or gardening.

What occupational therapy can do – for children and adults

Many of the people with dyspraxia interviewed for this book said they had had considerable help from occupational therapists once they had been diagnosed.

Aberdeen-based OT Therese Jackson explains what occupational therapists actually do.

> Basically, OTs help people carry out the activities of everyday living. This includes helping them to overcome the impact illness or injury has on their lives. Treatment is tailored to the individual and can involve improving their skills, adapting their activities, and/or altering their environment to enable them to carry out essential tasks in all areas of their lives, for example personal care, domestic life, work and leisure. We can't cure the condition but we can help people to cope in spite of it.

As well as people with dyspraxia, OTs often work with those recovering after accidents and stroke victims, helping to rehabilitate them so that they can become as independent as possible. An OT's job is, first of all, to assess exactly what the patient's problems are, and then to help them work out appropriate strategies to manage them.

Therese admits that it's not always easy to access OT help, especially for adults with dyspraxia.

'Paediatric OTs tend to say that adults are too old for them to work with but adult OTs tend to think of dyspraxia as a developmental problem,' she says.

A disturbing report published by the College of Occupational Therapists (COT) and the National Association of Paediatric OTs in July 2003 underlined what many parents of children with dyspraxia have found – that actually accessing OT help can be a major problem. The report found that children with dyspraxia have to wait an average of 46 weeks for an assessment, and that in some areas the wait can be as long as four years! Sheelagh Richards, Chief Executive of the COT, said, 'An unacceptable number of young people are getting a poor start in life because occupational therapy, and possibly other services, are unable to respond to their needs with sufficient priority.' (Contact details for COT are on page 89.)

If, as a patient, you are referred for OT help, the therapist will first of all assess exactly where your problems lie, and then work out how best to deal with them. For instance, even a task as apparently straightforward as making a cup of tea can be broken down into a sequence of smaller tasks – filling the kettle and switching it on, finding a mug, putting a teabag in the mug, pouring water into the mug, removing the teabag, getting milk from the fridge, pouring the right amount of milk into the mug, finding a spoon, adding sugar, stirring the tea and drinking it. In an ordinary household, this often has to be done at the same time as lots of other tasks – feeding the cat, getting the children's breakfasts, making sure they have the right books and games kit for school, perhaps answering the phone. All of which can be complicated and confusing for someone with dyspraxia, who may then miss out some vital part of the sequence like adding the teabag, or who may have difficulty pouring boiling water safely into a mug.

An OT will observe just what is going wrong for the patient. Can she not work out what she is supposed to do, or just how she is supposed to do it? Or can she do both, but somehow has trouble completing the task?

An assessment may include

- asking the patient to 'mime' the correct action – for example, pouring water from kettle to mug, stirring tea;
- imitating the movement carried out by the OT;
- being shown kettle, mug, spoon, etc., and asked to demonstrate how to use it;
- asking the patient to complete a more complex sequence – folding a piece of paper and putting it into an envelope, or spreading a slice of toast with both butter and jam.

Once the OT has worked out just where the problem lies she can offer the patient a series of exercises based on her individual needs, enabling her to carry out relevant everyday tasks more efficiently.

This can include things like breaking down each task into a sequence of smaller ones and practising each of them over and over, or showing the patient physically how to hold a cup, pour water, spread butter, button a cardigan, tie shoelaces, apply make-up or whatever is appropriate.

'The OT I saw asked me what I felt I needed help with,' says Elizabeth, who was in her late thirties, married and a mum by the time she was diagnosed.

I found many domestic tasks, like cooking and ironing, very difficult, so we concentrated on those. We went through everything one step at a time, leaving nothing to the imagination. I learned how best to set up an ironing board and which kind of iron suited me best. It turned out to be a cordless one. I was shown how to iron individual items like shirts and trousers and practised until I found it easier.

It was the same with cooking. My OT helped me to break everything down into a sequence of simple tasks which was really helpful. She also recommended suitable gadgets which made life easier for me, including a kettle-tipper which helped me to pour steadily. I had already found a potato-peeler I could use, but hadn't realized how many gadgets were available out there!

What seeing an educational or occupational psychologist can do – for children and adults

Many children and adults with dyspraxia are actually given their diagnosis by an educational (in the case of children) or occupational (in the case of adults) psychologist.

Madeleine Portwood is a Senior Educational Psychologist for Durham County Council and one of the country's leading experts on the condition. She has been interested in dyspraxia since 1988 when she was working with children with emotional and behavioural difficulties, many of whom had been excluded from school. She discovered that more than three-quarters of them had undiagnosed neurological developmental disorders, including dyspraxia.

'Accommodation must be made for these children,' she says.

The focus must be on normalization, as has already happened with dyslexia. Coping with the problems on a day-to-day basis is what really matters. In County Durham we have set up a Dyspraxia Service with specialist support at school and through parents.

What we have to do is integrate these children with their peer group, perhaps by pairing them, in school, with another, supportive child. If they are happy, they will work. If they are distressed and unhappy their teachers have to understand why this should be. The sort of help children are given in schools could include

- fine motor skills programmes to improve hand–eye co-ordination;
- triangular pencils which are easy to grip;
- sloping surfaces to write on;
- teachers writing down homework rather than expecting them to copy it down;
- colour-coding of books and files;
- no team-picking in PE lessons;
- the use of Dictaphones and so on.

In Durham, children with dyspraxia are now identified quickly and referred to the educational psychology service if they need help. A short course of therapy in a hospital clinic is all very well, but it's what happens in the rest of the child's life that counts. Parents, siblings and classmates can all help to make life easier – using a knife and fork, changing for PE, tape-recording homework or stories. Older children can be more selective about the activities they choose, picking those which don't require the same co-ordination. Early intervention for 4–6-year-olds saves so many problems later on. It's important that these children know they can achieve before their self-esteem is destroyed.

What speech therapy can do

Specialist speech therapist Pam Williams from the Nuffield Centre in London sees children from as young as 3 to teenagers.

'Most will already have been referred to a local speech therapist, but need extra help,' she comments.

Parents know there is something wrong. The child's speech may always have been unclear and has not improved. Some are really incomprehensible, even to their parents and to me! Obviously, if they start school with unclear speech they are likely to fall behind in reading, spelling and general literacy, and also become frustrated and withdrawn. Working with them I tend to concentrate on the actual production of sounds. For many children it can take a couple of years, but the long-term prognosis is good especially if developmental verbal dyspraxia is the only problem. Of course if they have additional difficulties with motor co-ordination or ADHD, treatment is more difficult.

Alan, who was diagnosed as an adult, found a speech therapist at his local hospital extremely helpful.

'Most of the specialists I contacted never wrote back, but this particular speech therapist happened to have a son with dyspraxia and jumped at the chance to see an adult with the same condition,' he says. 'I attended the hospital once a week for over a year. She went through everything, from correct breathing to how to accept compliments, in great detail, and this was a huge boost to my self-confidence.'

What counselling or psychotherapy can do

Many of those interviewed for this book had found counselling, psychotherapy and other 'talking' therapies helpful. This sort of treatment will not cure dyspraxia, but it *does* help with associated difficulties, like lack of self-confidence, relationship problems and even mild depression. Both children and adults can find it useful.

The fact that children and teenagers can suffer from mental health problems like anxiety and depression is not always understood. Children who have low self-esteem, who are 'picked on' or bullied because they are seen as 'different', who tend to be loners who have trouble making friends or keeping up with their peer group, are among those most likely to become anxious or depressed. Of course, not all children with dyspraxia come into these categories but many do. The organization Young Minds (contact details on

p. 93) has lots of information about how such children can be helped. This includes factsheets on subjects like depression, school phobia, school refusal and bullying, and information about counselling and psychotherapy services which are specifically for children and young people.

The British Association for Counselling and Psychotherapy (BACP) (contact details on p. 93) has free leaflets on choosing a counsellor or psychotherapist, and also on what sort of help you can expect from your sessions with them. Finding the right therapist is obviously crucial. You need someone with whom you feel safe and comfortable talking about your feelings and problems. The BACP has a list of therapists in all areas, together with details of any specialist training individuals may have had in, for instance, relationships counselling.

They point out that the aim of counselling and psychotherapy is *not* to tell clients what to do, but, as their Directory puts it, to 'guide us from feeling victims of circumstances, to feeling we have some control over our lives'. Some GPs can point you towards NHS counselling or psychotherapy, but it is more likely that you will have to pay for help. Fees do vary, and are sometimes negotiable for those who really can't afford to pay. Your first session with a therapist should be an exploratory one, giving both you and the therapist the chance to find out whether you can work together, if counselling is appropriate to your needs, and approximately how many sessions you are likely to need. Most sessions last from 50 minutes to an hour.

You might find descriptions of the various theoretical approaches to counselling and psychotherapy rather daunting at first. How can you work out whether Psychoanalysis, Primal Therapy, Adlerian Therapy or Neuro-Linguistic Programming is likely to help you? The BACP can tell you what all these terms mean, but they also say that, although some approaches seem to work better than others for specific difficulties, what really matters is the quality of the therapist. As an example, though, Cognitive Behavioural Therapy (CBT) has been found effective in the treatment of both stress-related ailments and depression, each of which can affect those struggling to manage dyspraxia. The idea of CBT is to modify the self-defeating thought patterns that can lead to both anxiety and depression. Clients are taught ways to change their thoughts and expectations, partly by the use of relaxation techniques and also by practising new behaviours.

The Dyspraxia Foundation's Adult Support Group can also provide information about local sources of help.

8

'Is There an Alternative?'

Because there is, as yet, no cure for dyspraxia, many of those affected by the condition look outside mainstream medicine for support. The Dyspraxia Foundation only recognizes mainstream therapies like physiotherapy, occupational therapy and speech and language therapy under the NHS or in the private sector. While complementary therapies undoubtedly offer benefits in some areas, like stress reduction, the Dyspraxia Foundation neither endorses nor discredits any individual complementary therapy or treatment. The Foundation recommends that anyone considering any kind of complementary therapy should:

- request independent evidence that the therapy has been thoroughly researched and validated – for instance, that papers have been published in reputable peer-reviewed journals;
- ask for the names and contact details of other people who have had the treatment, and follow them up;
- enquire whether the therapist is accredited with the appropriate professional body and check that they are;
- check with the British Medical Association to find out whether the therapy is recognized by the medical profession.

Claims that any 'complementary' treatment is a miracle cure – especially if it involves handing over large sums of money – should always be taken with a pinch of salt. It is also sensible to choose a form of therapy you feel comfortable with and a therapist you trust and feel that you can work with. Premises – whether a clinic or a private house – should always be clean and comfortable. Don't be afraid to ask questions. Try to discover whether your therapist has treated people with dyspraxia before and what kind of results she obtained. Be realistic, also, about the results you expect. Most complementary therapists will not even claim to be able to 'cure' dyspraxia, but they could help with attendant problems like self-esteem, relationship difficulties, anxiety or depression.

There are private clinics and institutes offering specialized treatment for children with developmental disorders. These include the Chester-based Institute for Neuro-Physiological Psychology (INPP), and the Dyslexia, Dyspraxia and Attention Disorder Treatment (DDAT) Centre, based in Kenilworth but with six other centres around Britain, whose exercise programmes are said to be effective in improving the condition.

DDAT Centres

The DDAT Centres were set up by a millionaire businessman whose own daughter was severely dyslexic. Their approach is based on the theory that developmental disorders like dyslexia and dyspraxia are caused by delayed development of the cerebellum, the part of the brain which controls motor skills, balance and co-ordination. An assessment at one of the DDAT Centres is followed by a personally tailored programme of exercises to be done morning and evening for up to a year. Progress visits to the Centre are made every six weeks. Once the programme is complete the exercises can be discontinued, but patients often continue to make progress. A course of treatment at one of the DDAT Centres costs around £1,500.

Clinical trials on the DDAT approach have been carried out by Professor David Reynolds of Exeter University, with encouraging results.

'We have carried out a number of studies comparing children who had followed the DDAT treatment with those who had not,' he says.

Some of the children we have looked at have dyslexia, some have dyspraxia, some have ADHD, and many have combinations of all three disorders. It's possible that different symptom complexes will produce different results over time.

Basically, we have found that children who started the programme 18 months to two years behind their peers in reading have caught up after treatment, and the effect holds for a year at least. Now we are trying to understand the variations in results between individuals. We are collecting data about family background and environmental factors as well. We plan to divide the children into groups and look at how successfully the programme treats those with dyslexia, dyspraxia and a combination of conditions.

The Dyspraxia Foundation points out that these are only preliminary results and that only time will tell whether this form of treatment will be as successful, in the long term, as established exercise programmes such as those devised by physiotherapists. Many of the exercises in the DDAT programme – marching on the spot, throwing and catching bean-bags, 'crossing the midline' – are similar to those recommended by physios. However, Professor Reynolds says that the emphasis is slightly different, focusing on 'eye tracking' for speed and accuracy, and 'vestibular function' which affects balance. The emphasis seems to be on the visual, rather than just on the physical, and the exercises, which are tailored for each individual, are rather more sensitive and sophisticated. (Contact details for the DDAT and INPP clinics are on p. 96.)

The INPP

The INPP was set up in 1975 by psychologist Peter Blythe and in the last five or ten years its approach has become more widely accepted. It is based on the theory that all babies are born with what the INPP calls 'primitive reflexes' which are replaced, as the baby develops, by 'postural reflexes'. As the reflexes mature, proper hand–eye co-ordination, motor and language skills are able to develop. The problem for children with dyspraxia is that they retain the primitive reflexes. Treatment involves a series of stereotyped exercises to be repeated every day in order to develop the postural reflexes.

'Patients are still not referred to us by GPs, perhaps because we are not labelled "medical", but we have done a great deal of research and many of our programmes are used in schools,' comments Sally Goddard Blythe, who is also a psychologist and has published a number of papers on the work of the Institute.

> The tests we use to assess the people who come to us are from mainstream medicine and the exercises we recommend are similar to those prescribed by occupational therapists. We never claim to cure dyspraxia but if people fit the right profile, we can help them. That includes many dyspraxics as well as dyslexics and those with attention deficit disorder (ADD), panic and anxiety disorders.

The underlying problem is immaturity of the central nervous system. In order to read well you need ocular skills. In order to write well you need hand–eye co-ordination. If you have an underlying problem at a reflex level, it will affect all your motor skills as well as your balance and posture. We have a simple but comprehensive developmental screening questionnaire covering family history, pregnancy, birth and early development. If a patient ticks more than seven 'yes' answers on this, we can probably help him.

The exercises we prescribe are based on normal infant movement patterns – the vocabulary of early movement, if you like – while those prescribed by physios and OTs tend to start at a later, 'crawling' level. Our exercises are designed to stimulate the development of later, postural reflexes. Children need to do them for five or ten minutes a day, at home, for about a year, and we review their progress at 6–8 weekly intervals.

We have already trained about 2,000 teachers to use the programme and results have been very encouraging. In one programme at a Carlisle primary school, children who were drawing at a 4/5-year-old level were drawing at a 9/10-year-old level at the end of the year. We are currently involved in setting up a similar programme, involving 800 children, in Northern Ireland.

A full programme, including assessment, tests and follow-up appointments at the INPP clinic, will cost in the region of £800–900.

A change of diet

Nutrition therapy is on the border between complementary and mainstream medicine. The idea of dietary manipulation as a cure for behavioural problems in children is not a new one. Back in the 1970s, American scientists were suggesting that a diet of junk food, high in chemical additives as well as saturated fat, sugar and salt, could contribute to crime and delinquency. Youths in young offenders' institutions behaved better when they were fed on a healthier and more natural diet. Conditions like ADHD, which are known to be related to dyspraxia, can sometimes be helped by a change of diet. It's true that some experts are inclined to dismiss the dietary approach and prefer to treat ADHD children with drugs like Ritalin, but some parents do find that a more natural, additive-free diet improves their children's behaviour.

Additives are only part of the story. As long ago as 1981, the Sussex-based Hyperactive Children's Support Group (HCSG) was recommending the use of essential fatty acid (EFA) supplements, in the form of evening primrose oil, in the diets of hyperactive children. Recent studies at Oxford University adding fish oil to the diets of children with ADHD have confirmed that it can be helpful. American research studies subsequently suggested that the problem may not be that these children are not getting enough EFAs in their diet, but rather that they are unable to metabolize them for some reason. Many children with ADHD are also found to be deficient in minerals like zinc and magnesium. Sally Bunday, founder of the HCSG, feels that a holistic approach to the nutrition of hyperactive children works best. In other words, they may need additional vitamins and mineral supplements, notably zinc, magnesium and Vitamin B6, in addition to essential fatty acids.

'Not enough research has been done into the effect of EFAs on children with dyspraxia and dyslexia,' she comments.

> However, parents do tell us that a change of diet improves their children's co-ordination. Their handwriting improves and they are better able to cope with activities like riding a bicycle. Of course, we have no way of knowing whether this is a direct effect of the diet changes or whether it is because their concentration has also improved.

Studies on dyslexia at Surrey University resulted in similar findings. Particularly for children who have ADHD as well as dyspraxia, a look at diet seems worthwhile. Information can be obtained from ADHD support groups (contact details on p. 89).

There is actually some recent evidence that diet, and specifically Omega-3 and Omega-6 fatty acid supplements, may indeed have a part to play in the effective management of dyspraxia in some people. Durham Local Education Authority, in association with the Dyslexia Research Trust, carried out a study of 111 children of primary-school age with dyslexia, dyspraxia and related conditions, in order to find out whether these supplements can help. The supplement used was Equazen eye q™ which is a blend of high-grade marine fish oil and evening primrose oil, with added Vitamin E.

Some of the results were mentioned in Lord Winston's BBC-TV programme *The Human Mind*, screened in October 2003. The children were assessed both before and after taking the supplements, for IQ, distractibility, organizational skills, manual dexterity, ball skills and balance, as well as reading, spelling, handwriting, memory and excitability/hyperactivity. The research was carried out under randomized, double-blind, placebo-controlled conditions. The children took six tablets a day and were then asked to blow through a tube to provide breath samples. These were then tested for a gas called *ethane*, which is normally produced as fatty acids break down in the body. The test identifies the children who use up the fatty acids more quickly than normal, and who could therefore benefit most from supplements.

Some of the results were very impressive, with both teachers and parents reporting changes in children's behaviour and attitudes in weeks. Reading, memory and concentration all seemed to improve. After three months of taking supplements, one child's reading age increased by an impressive four years, with an increase of two years reported in some of the other children. It has been suggested that fatty acids may assist in building up the myelin sheath around neurons as well as the neurons themselves.

It is also possible that fatty acids make it easier for electrical signals in the brain to 'jump' the synaptic gap between neurons.

HUFAs

Why should Omega-3 and Omega-6 oils have this effect? These are known as highly unsaturated essential fatty acids (HUFAs), and are obtainable from the diet – in oily fish such as herring, haddock, mackerel and salmon, unprocessed fish oils, linseed and walnut oils, pumpkin seeds and green leafy vegetables. It has long been known that these HUFAs help to protect the heart, boost the immune system and improve skin conditions like eczema. (Inuit peoples, who have a high HUFA intake, have a death rate from heart disease which is only about one-tenth that of most Western countries.)

It is also now known that these HUFAs are essential for normal brain development and functioning. Lower than average levels of HUFAs have been found in blood samples of children with ADHD. About a third to a half of the human brain and a proportion of the retina is actually made up of essential fatty acids. Sadly, modern Western diets tend to be deficient in these vital nutrients and contain too much saturated fat (in meat and dairy products) and trans fatty acids (in margarine, processed foods, crisps and biscuits). To make things more complicated, the optimum ratio of Omega-3 to Omega-6 fatty acids in the diet has not yet been agreed. In some modern diets the ratio can be as high as 100:1. Inuit diets produce a ratio of 2.5:1 and Mediterranean diets a ratio of 1:6. Research suggests that the combined benefits are greater than those of the oils taken individually. Researchers are also still working on ways to identify which patients will benefit most from this kind of supplement.

Mary Colley, of the Adult Dyspraxia Support Group, says that some members do find these supplements helpful although there is little research to date on what they can do for adults. The Durham LEA/Dyslexia Research Trust study referred to above found that in about one-third of the children, the problem seemed to be metabolic and not neurological – in other words, their bodies had a problem breaking down the fatty acids into a form that they could use.

Fish oil supplements – or even simply eating more oily fish – seems a promising area for research studies, but supplements don't benefit everyone, as Fiona found out when she gave them to her 13-year-old daughter Kerry.

'I was never really convinced I was giving her anything more useful than cod-liver oil,' she says ruefully. 'Kerry hated it and I was told that if it hadn't improved her condition after a certain length of time, then it probably wasn't right for her. As far as we could tell, it didn't affect her at all.'

Fiona says she is open-minded about complementary therapies.

'If Kerry agrees, it's not invasive, has nice people attached to it, it does not upset her and we can just about afford it, we'll give it a try,' she says.

Most of the techniques Fiona tried were useful for stress relief and helped Kerry to sleep but didn't have any measurable effect on the dyspraxia.

For example I wouldn't say cranial osteopathy was any real help, but the practitioner was a really nice man and it was very relaxing. We also saw a therapist who produced a special personally designed audio tape for Kerry which was supposed to be on the right frequency for her brain. She used to go to sleep listening to it . . . but whether we would have got the same effect with an ordinary tape of New Age-type music, I have no way of knowing. That same therapist had been trained in 'neuro-developmental therapy', which involved Kerry having to practise a programme of very repetitive movements. Unfortunately we moved house and could no longer get to the therapist or we might have persevered with that one as it could have had a concrete measurable effect.

I think the 'therapy' which has actually benefited Kerry most is horse-riding. At first, we had a problem getting her accepted in her local Riding for the Disabled group, as she doesn't look disabled, but eventually they did take her. Kerry loves animals and now, after six years, she can actually swing her leg over the horse in a way she couldn't when she started. She manages to turn right and turn left much better on horseback, too. As well as developing a relationship with the horses, it has done a lot for her social integration. She has always had her birthday parties at the stables and mixes happily with the other kids.

Research into the possibilities of dietary supplementation is ongoing. It goes without saying that people with dyspraxia, like everyone else, should try to keep their strength up and their stress levels down by eating a balanced, healthy diet, which means one low in animal fats and sugars and rich in fruit and vegetables. The right food can affect your mood and combat depression, according to nutritionist and psychologist Patrick Holford, who recommends

- avoiding sugar and sugary snacks, which only give a short-term energy boost and lead to wildly fluctuating blood-sugar levels and hence mood swings;
- reducing the use of stimulants like tea, coffee, chocolate and cigarettes;
- increasing your intake of nutrient-rich foods like fruit and vegetables, wholefoods, wheatgerm, seeds, poultry, tofu and beans;
- eating oily fish three times a week.

A sensible exercise programme has been proved to lift mild depression. Practising a form of exercise you really enjoy – anything from swimming or golf to brisk walking or horse-riding – can help to release endorphins, the brain's feel-good hormones.

Improving your co-ordination

There is also anecdotal evidence that some people with dyspraxia benefit from those therapies which are actually designed to improve physical co-ordination – like the Alexander Technique, yoga and Pilates.

The Alexander Technique was developed by an Australian actor, Frederick Matthias Alexander, at the end of the nineteenth century. He was having trouble with his voice during Shakespearean recitals, and after looking at himself carefully in a mirror he realized that he was using his body wrongly, tensing his neck muscles and pulling his head back. Eventually he devised a technique which enabled him to establish new patterns of balance and co-ordination throughout his whole body, which resulted in a better alignment of his head, neck, back and torso.

Since balance and co-ordination are often a problem in dyspraxia, it sounds as though the Alexander Technique might be just the right method for those who have the condition. Alexander teachers do not claim to be able to cure any specific condition or medical disorder. The Technique is taught on an individual basis and there are no set exercises or movements as there are with yoga or Pilates. Those who have studied the Technique say that they have more energy, are calmer, more relaxed and suffer from fewer ailments like insomnia, stress and breathing problems.

Doctor and Alexander teacher Miriam Wohl emphasizes that although clinical trials have not yet been carried out to explore whether the Alexander Technique can benefit those with dyspraxia, her own medical and physiological knowledge, plus a hundred years of accumulated Alexander teaching experience, indicate that it can be helpful. (Contact details are on page 97.)

Learning the Alexander Technique is like having driving lessons for your own human vehicle. You learn how to 'drive' yourself as well as possible – in other words you learn the quality of thought and muscle tone required to carry out the activities of daily living. You are working with a less-than-perfect nervous system in a condition such as dyspraxia. Learning and applying the Alexander Technique will enable you to make the most of your available neurological ability and use it in the best possible way.

Pilates

Pilates is a system of exercises devised just after the First World War by a German émigré to America called Joseph Pilates. It originally became popular with dancers in New York and has evolved over the years. Those studying Pilates say it helps to achieve better balance, muscle co-ordination and graceful movement.

Lynne Robinson is the author of many books and videos on Pilates and says that when she took it up she suffered from poor balance and co-ordination herself.

> I don't think I have ever taught anyone with dyspraxia, but Pilates is about re-educating people in good movement skills. We work a lot on body awareness, how you position your body when doing the exercises, and the movements are very precise. The process of re-education is the same whether I am working with someone with poor co-ordination or an elite athlete. Learning a physical skill or set of movements is amazing mind–body training. Many Pilates teachers are also physiotherapists so anyone with dyspraxia might benefit from working with them.

(Contact details are on p. 96.)

Some people with dyspraxia report that they find yoga beneficial, not least because it's a form of exercise which is absolutely non-competitive and not, as is sometimes thought, about contorting one's body into impossible poses. The word 'yoga' comes from the Sanskrit for 'union', and yoga is designed to promote union between mind and body. As well as increasing bodily strength and suppleness, yoga helps to calm the mind and relax the body. Yoga teacher Maya Sendell, who has worked with members of the Dyspraxia Foundation's Adult Support Group, says that yoga helps people to feel comfortable about thinking with their body, as well as their mind.

'It is a very accessible therapy, and not intimidating,' she says, 'especially because you don't have to worry about whether you are "good at it". I would recommend working in small classes with an accredited teacher.'

Relaxation

Just as exercise-based therapies may help with co-ordination problems, it's also possible that the many complementary treatments which aid relaxation may improve the emotional state of those with dyspraxia. Massage and aromatherapy are always soothing. Aroma-therapists recommend essential oils – either in baths, inhaled, used for massage or as room fragrances – as a way of treating all kinds of emotional states. For example, Cedarwood, Chamomile, Clary Sage, Geranium, Juniper, Lavender, Marjoram and Tangerine are all recommended for treating general stress. For a more detailed and personal analysis, it's best to consult a qualified aromatherapist (contact details on p. 96).

Bach Flower Remedies

At the turn of the last century, Dr Edward Bach, a consultant bacteriologist and homoeopath, developed a range of natural, plant-based remedies designed to promote not just physical but also emotional health and well-being. The 38 Bach Flower Remedies were each devised to deal with specific emotional states and circumstances. For instance, Walnut is used in periods of transition such as adolescence and the 'change of life' as well as for people adjusting to new beginnings or relationships. Larch is used to treat those lacking in self-confidence and Sweet Chestnut for those who feel they have reached the limit of their endurance.

Bach Flower Remedies are completely safe and can be used alongside other complementary or conventional treatments. One of the best-known is Bach Rescue Remedy, obtainable in homoeopathic pharmacies and health-food shops. It's a combination of five Flower Remedies (Rock Rose for terror, Impatiens for irritability, Clematis for absent-mindedness, Star of Bethlehem for feelings after trauma, Cherry Plum for fear of losing control) and is intended to comfort and reassure in any kind of stressful situation – from examinations to job interviews. It can also be used on children and animals (contact details on p. 95).

9

What about the Future?

Ask anyone with dyspraxia what they would like to see happen in the future and the answer comes in one word: AWARENESS. Things are improving for people – and especially children – with developmental disorders, but only slowly. Dyspraxia is now roughly where dyslexia was twenty or thirty years ago. Some health professionals and members of the general public know what it is but many still don't.

In the 'bad old days' children with dyslexia were just thought to be 'backward' when it came to reading. Children with ADHD were just considered to be badly behaved, naughty or uncontrollable and it was generally assumed that it was their parents' fault! It took a long time and considerable campaigning before it was accepted that such children actually had a recognized and diagnosable medical condition, and that their problems were very real and not just the result of 'middle-class neurotic mums making a fuss' – as one mother described it.

As Professor David Reynolds of Exeter University admits,

Originally, dyslexia was just thought to be middle-class reading failure, and there are still some people who believe that. However, today's research in this area is tending more towards physiological explanations for these conditions, rather than environmental ones. It may be that some people have physiological or genetic reasons for developing dyspraxia and then some environmental factors trigger it off.

Research is increasingly looking at the brains of people with dyspraxia, rather than their backgrounds, to explain exactly why and how the condition occurs.

Research psychologist Margaret Cousins is hoping to continue her work and says that future researchers will be hoping to build up a bigger picture of what exactly causes the varied symptoms of the condition.

'We will need to set up complicated research studies involving lots of children,' she says.

We need to find out whether groups of children with the same symptoms have the same underlying cause. We still don't know whether all the developmental disorders are the result of atypical brain development. It's a confusing field for research because some researchers are studying balance, some are studying timing, and many, of course, are focusing on dyslexia, ADHD or autism rather than dyspraxia by itself.

It is known that there is an association between low birthweight and prematurity and dyspraxia – but just as not all premature babies grow up to have dyspraxia, not all of those with dyspraxia were premature babies! There is a lot we still don't know although researchers are slowly building up a wider picture.

No drugs are available to treat dyspraxia at the moment or in the foreseeable future. In the meantime, treatment is still largely a matter of developing strategies to enable children and adults to cope with everyday life. How much help individual patients get is still a matter of luck.

'We need to encourage more mainstream services for people with dyspraxia through Local Education Authorities and Health Services,' says educational psychologist Madeleine Portwood.

At the moment, waiting lists for physio and occupational therapy are far too long. Structured PE lessons in schools could help many children, and then the small number who actually need specialist help could be referred on. Motor programmes in PE will always help with co-ordination but co-ordination is only part of the problem. We need to address children's learning difficulties – with things like handwriting – and their social problems with their peers as well.

I would like to see a normalization of the condition. The most important thing is how dyspraxia affects children's learning and family relationships. More opportunities for trained adults to support children in the classroom, more visual and interactive learning so that children don't have to record everything by hand. Computers aren't a complete answer as these children's keyboard skills are not always that good either.

I would also like to see more attention paid to informing other children about the condition. Instead of teaching dyspraxic children how to cope with the stress of being left out or bullied, why not remove the source of the stress by educating their peer group to support them?

'I would like the Health Service and Education Authorities to provide practical information that is available to any parent, anywhere,' says Dr Amanda Kirby from the Dyscovery Centre in Cardiff.

This could include ideas to help children with dressing, writing, bottom-wiping, using scissors, playing ball games – everything dyspraxic children need.

I would like to see every affected family have a keyworker, to help them negotiate their way around services, and link the process so no one misses out.

I would like to see IT used to provide staff training across different services so that we are all singing from the same hymn sheet.

I would also like to see baseline screening to identify the children in schools who are having problems.

As far as research is concerned, there is a lot that we need to find out about the causes of dyspraxia, which parts of the brain are affected and which genes. I'd like to see more research into different treatments and how they should be implemented. The development of computerized screening tools to identify affected children, using things like webcams, for distance assessments would be very useful.

Professor Neil Marlow of Queen's Medical Centre in Nottingham says that medical technology is moving forward all the time, offering interesting new techniques in areas like brain scanning, to give researchers a better idea of what actually happens in the brains of people with dyspraxia.

'Functional Magnetic Resonance Imaging gives us a measure of how the brain organizes itself,' he says. 'However this is quite a difficult area to study, especially in childhood, as it involves children lying still for quite a long time, which isn't easy for those with dyspraxia or ADHD.'

The Dyspraxia Foundation – future plans

As well as spreading the word about dyspraxia and offering support through local groups and their national newsletter to affected families, the Dyspraxia Foundation has all sorts of plans for the future.

'We are helping to set up a Government all-party working group, looking at the issues surrounding dyspraxia,' says spokeswoman Eleanor Howes.

> We have already started this moving, with a meeting at the House of Commons on our first National Dyspraxia Awareness Day in July 2003. A number of MPs have expressed an interest.
>
> We are also planning to do our own research, looking at waiting times for assessment and treatment of dyspraxia around the UK. We will be looking at the impact on the family, and the implications for the child.
>
> We shall be building on the success of the first National Awareness Day to raise the level of awareness, enabling all those affected to reach their full potential in life. We're working with Primary Health Care Trusts and other organizations to improve the services available.
>
> We are organizing a two-day conference in Birmingham for all professionals working in the field. We are also forming links with a variety of support and information groups around the UK covering the spectrum of special needs.

What would campaigners like to see? Mary Colley of the Adult Support Group has no hesitation.

'I would like to see dyspraxia *recognized* in adults,' she says firmly.

> Too many people, even some of the so-called experts, seem to believe it's a condition that you grow out of. Those of us in the Adult Support Group know that just isn't true. Treatment should be available for us on the NHS without us having to fight for it and without the ridicule some of us have to face. After all, no one expects people with dyslexia or Asperger's Syndrome to grow out of it, so why should we?

I would also like to see the various organizations working for those with dyslexia, dyspraxia, ADHD and Asperger's working together because we have a lot in common.

Mary has just started DANDA, a new group focusing its energies entirely on adults with developmental disorders – dyspraxia, dyslexia, ADHD, Asperger's and all related conditions. Many of the people in the Adult Support Group have more than one of them.

'We plan to apply for charitable status once the group is up and running,' she says.

The idea of DANDA is that it should focus on adults alone and be run by adult members for adult members. An independent group should give us all choices about our own future and give us a proper voice as adults. The problems dyspraxia causes don't go away when you are 18 or 25.

The parents of children with dyspraxia also have plenty of ideas about how life could be improved for them – for example:

- shorter waits between diagnosis and treatment – waits of a year to 18 months are not uncommon;
- more information on special needs in ordinary teacher training, including more awareness of hidden disabilities;
- recognition that some children learn in a different way, and that this doesn't mean they are wrong, just different.

Meg, whose 13-year-old daughter Chloe has just transferred from a mainstream secondary school to a school for children with moderate learning difficulties, feels that many schools have a long way to go before they are able to offer children with dyspraxia the kind of education which really meets their needs.

Chloe's mainstream school did what it could, but in a class of thirty children it's terribly difficult for the teacher to give each child exactly the right individual attention. Now, at her special school, Chloe is in a class of eight and is valued for what she can do, as well as learning life skills like cooking that she didn't have before. Many schools do try, I know, but in a secondary school where children have a different set of teachers every year, it's hard for all of them to understand exactly what an individual child's needs are. Some teachers still seem to think children with dyspraxia are lazy, or not trying.

Chloe had an especially hard time with her PE teacher and used to get terribly upset before games lessons because allowances were just not made for her disability. Dyspraxia *is* a disability and should be recognized as one.

Pam, whose son Jon's statement of special needs has not been reviewed for almost six years, says that what would improve life for her, and the other families in her local dyspraxia support group, is for medical and educational help to be available locally, without parents having to fight for it!

'I hear of two- and three-year waits for occupational therapy and funding for special-needs support at school being cut and it makes me so angry,' she comments. 'So many parents don't know where to go for help or what help is available and it isn't made easy for them.'

Some experts are even questioning the value of the 'dyspraxia' label, although they recognize that parents and individuals always want to know exactly what is wrong.

'We put a great deal of pressure on our children to perform – and to conform,' comments Professor Neil Marlow of Queen's Medical Centre in Nottingham.

We give them a lot of complex tasks to do, and when they fail we might be a bit too ready to label them abnormal. It has been pointed out that there is no such thing as 'abnormal' if you are growing up in Papua New Guinea. In a society like that you are just given jobs to do which are suited to your abilities, rather than being judged because you think and behave differently. Perhaps the best way to manage dyspraxia is to learn to play to people's successes, rather than their failures.

10

Useful Addresses

Help with dyspraxia and other developmental disorders

Dyspraxia Connexion
21 Birchdale Avenue
Hucknall
Nottingham NG15 6DL

Tel: 0115 963 2220
website <www.dysf.fsnet.co.uk>
email <notts@dysf.fsnet.co.uk>

Dyspraxia E-list
<dyspraxia@yahoogroups.com>

Dyspraxia Foundation
8 West Alley
Hitchin
Herts SG5 1EG

Telephone Helpline: 01462 454986
website <www.dyspraxiafoundation.org.uk>
email <dyspraxia@dyspraxiafoundation.org.uk>

Dyspraxia Foundation Adult Support Group
c/o Mary Colley
46 Westbere Road
London NW2 3RU

Tel: 020 7435 7891
email <adultdyspraxia@pmcolley.freeserve.co.uk>
or <mary@pmcolley.freeserve.co.uk>

British Dyslexia Association
98 London Road
Reading RG1 5AU

Telephone Helpline 0118 966 8271
website <www.bda-dyslexia.org.uk>
email <admin@dyslexia-bda.demon.co.uk>

Chartered Society of Physiotherapy
14 Bedford Row
London WC1R 4ED

Tel: 020 7306 6666
website <www.csp.org.uk>
email <csp@csphysio.org.uk>

College of Occupational Therapists
106–114 Borough High Street
London SE1 1LB

Tel: 020 7357 6480
website <www.cot.org.uk>

Dyscovery Centre
4A Church Road
Whitchurch
Cardiff CF14 2DZ

Tel: 029 2062 8222
website <www.dyscovery.co.uk>
email <dyscoverycentre@btclick.com>

Hyperactive Children's Support Group
71 Whyke Lane
Chichester
West Sussex PO19 7PD

Tel: 01243 551313
website <www.hacsg.org.uk>
email <contact@hacsg.org.uk>

The Lee Medical Practice
Blaire House
Denham Green Lane
Denham
Bucks UB9 5LQ

Tel: 01895 835144
email <michele@leemedical.fsnet.co.uk>

National Autistic Society
393 City Road
London EC1V 1NG

Telephone Helpline: 0870 600 8585
website <www.nas.org.uk>
email <nas@nas.org.uk>

Royal College of Speech and Language Therapists
2 White Hart Yard
London SE1 1NX

Tel: 020 7378 1200
website <www.rcslt.org>
email <postmaster@rcslt.org>

Early years education

National Childminding Association
8 Masons Hill
Bromley
Kent BR2 9EY

Telephone Information Line 0800 169 4486
website <www.ncma.org.uk>
email <info@ncma.org.uk>

Pre-School Learning Alliance
National Centre
69 King's Cross Road
London WC1X 9LL

Tel: 020 7833 0991
website <www.pre-school.org.uk>
email <pla@pre-school.org.uk>

Step Forward Publishing
The Coach House
Cross Road
Milverton
Leamington Spa
Warwicks CV32 5PB

Tel: 01926 420046
website <www.practicalpreschool.com>
email <enquiries@practicalpreschool.com>

Publishes *Practical Pre-School* magazine and leaflets about early years education, including special-needs education.

School-age children

Childline
45 Folgate Street
London E1 6GL

Telephone Helpline 0800 1111
(Admin.) 020 7650 3200
website <www.childline.org.uk>

Connexions Direct
Tel: 080 800 13-2-19
website <www.connexions-direct.com>

Department for Education and Skills Publications Centre
PO Box 5050
Sherwood Park
Annersley
Nottingham NG15 0DJ

Tel: 0845 602 2260
website <www.dfes.gov.uk/sen>
email <dfes@prolog.uk.com>

The Home School
46 Alkham Road
London N16 7AA

Tel: 020 8806 6965
email <homeskool@alkham.demon.co.uk>

Inclusive Solutions
49 Northcliffe Avenue
Nottingham NG3 6DA

Tel: 0115 955 6045 or 0115 960 5071
website <www.inclusive-solutions.com>
email <inclusive.solutions@ntlworld.com>

National Pyramid Trust
84 Uxbridge Road
London W13 8RA

Tel: 020 8579 5108
website <www.nptrust.org.uk>
email <enquiries@nptrust.co.uk>

Parents for Inclusion
Unit 2
70 South Lambeth Road
London SW8 1RL

Telephone Helpline 0800 652 3145
website <www.parentsforinclusion.org>
email <info@parentsforinclusion.org>

SKILL
Chapter House
18–20 Crucifix Lane
London SE1 3JW

Telephone Helpline 0800 328 5050
website <www.skill.org.uk>
email <skill@skill.org.uk>

The National Bureau for students with disabilities.

Young Minds
102–108 Clerkenwell Road
London EC1M 5SA

Parents' Information Line: 0800 018 2138
Tel: 020 7336 8445
website <www.youngminds.org.uk>
email <enquiries@youngminds.org.uk>

Adult life

Benefits Enquiry Line (for people with disabilities)
0800 88 22 00

British Association for Counselling and Psychotherapy
BACP House
35–37 Albert Street
Rugby
Warwicks CV21 2SG

Tel: 0870 443 5252
website <www.bacp.co.uk>
email <bacp@bacp.co.uk>

BSM (British School of Motoring)
Telephone Helpline 08457 276 276
website <www.bsm.co.uk/mobility/index.html>
email via website

Department for Transport MAVIS scheme
Crowthorne Business Estate
Old Wokingham Road
Crowthorne
Berkshire RG45 6XD

Tel: 01344 661000
website <www.dft.gov.uk/access/mavis>

Disability Rights Commission
DRC Helpline
Freepost MID02164
Stratford-upon-Avon CV37 9BR

Tel: 0845 762 2633
website <www.drc-gb.org>

Disabled Living Foundation
380–384 Harrow Road
London W9 2HU

Telephone Helpline 0845 130 9177
website <www.dlf.org.uk>
email <advice@dlf.org.uk>

Driving Standards Agency
Stanley House
56 Talbot Street
Nottingham NG1 5GU

Tel: 0115 901 2500
website <www.dsa.gov.uk>
email <customer.services@dsa.qsi.gov.uk>

Employers' Forum on Disability
Nutmeg House
60 Gainsford Street
London SE1 2NY

Tel: 020 7403 3020
website <www.employers-forum.co.uk>
email <website.enquiries@employers-forum.co.uk>

Keep Able
Telephone Helpline 0870 520 2122

Stores and mail-order service for disability aids.

Mental Health Foundation
83 Victoria Street
London SW1H 0HW

Tel: 020 7802 0300
website <www.mentalhealth.org.uk>
email <mhf@mhf.org.uk>

MIND (National Association for Mental Health)
Granta House
15–19 Broadway
Stratford
London E15 4BQ

Telephone Helpline 0845 766 0163
website <www.mind.org.uk>
email <contact@mind.org.uk>

RADAR
12 City Forum
250 City Road
London EC1V 8AF

Tel: 020 7250 3222
website <www.radar.org.uk>
email <radar@radar.co.uk>

Ways and Means
Nottingham Rehab Supplies
Findel House
Excelsior Road
Ashby Park
Ashby de la Zouch
Leics LE65 1NG
Telephone Helpline 0845 606 0911
website <www.nrs-uk.co.uk>
email <nrscustomerservice@nrs-uk.co.uk>

Has a catalogue of disability aids.

Is there an alternative?

Bach Flower Remedies
The Bach Centre
Mount Vernon
Bakers Lane
Sotwell
Oxfordshire OX10 0PZ

Tel: 01491 834678
website <www.bachcentre.com>

Body Control Pilates
6 Langley Street
London WC2H 9JA

Tel: 020 7379 3734
website <www.bodycontrol.co.uk>
email <info@bodycontrol.co.uk>

British Wheel of Yoga
25 Jermyn Street
Sleaford
Lincs NG34 7RU

Tel: 01529 306851
website <www.bwy.org.uk>
email <office@bwy.org.uk>

DDAT (Dore Achievement Centres)
Camden House
Warwick Road
Kenilworth
Warwickshire CV8 1TH

Tel: 0870 737 0017
website <www.ddat.co.uk>
email <info@dorecentres.co.uk>

Institute for Neuro-Physiological Psychology (INPP)
Warwick House
4 Stanley Place
Chester CH1 2LU

Tel: 01244 311414
website <www.inpp.org.uk>
email <mail@inpp.org.uk>

International Federation of Professional Aromatherapists
82 Ashby Road
Hinckley
Leicestershire LE10 1SN

Tel: 01455 637987
website <www.ifparoma.org>
email <admin@ifparoma.org>

Society of Teachers of the Alexander Technique
1st Floor
Linton House
39–51 Highgate Road
London NW5 1RS

Tel: 0845 230 7828
website <www.stat.org.uk>

Appendix

Twelve Top Tips on Coping with Dyspraxia – for Children and Adults

1 Take it a day at a time.
2 Calm parents, structure in everyday life and a high level of predictability all seem to help dyspraxic children.
3 Make sure you know which problems are caused by your child's dyspraxia and which by his/her own personality.
4 Improve your child's self-esteem by finding an 'island of competence' – something your child does well, or is especially interested in.
5 Tell other people at school or work what the problems are and how you can be helped to cope with them. Teachers, bosses and workmates can't help if they don't understand what's wrong.
6 Remember there are ways round most difficulties. Having said that, accept there are things you just can't do. Concentrate on the things you *can* do – and do well.
7 Don't expect children with dyspraxia to learn from what they see. Instead, practise doing it with them.
8 Don't wait until they are ready to learn. Dyspraxic children never are!
9 Computer skills can be a godsend, especially for teenagers.
10 Remember that you are the expert on your child as you are with them 24 hours a day, not the 20 minutes or so they spend with the doctor.
11 Join a local support group and meet other parents, who can often offer invaluable tips to help you cope with everyday life – things like replacing buttons with Velcro fasteners and colour-coding homework files.
12 Always, always try to see the funny side.

Index